# What Others Are Saying

Dear Readers:

In her book, *Rainbows After the Storms*, you have the joy of meeting one of the most delightful women I have had the privilege of meeting and calling my friend. Julia Widlacki radiates joy, love, encouragement, and humility. She brings to life and demonstrates the surprising instruction of James, who writes in his letter: "Consider it pure joy, my brothers, whenever you face trials of many kinds, Because you know that the testing of your faith develops perseverance and perseverance must finish its work so that you may be mature and complete, not lacking anything" (Biblical Reference: James 1:2–4).

Always, whether visiting her at home, checking in on her in a hospital room, or talking in the church house, my wife and I have walked away refreshed, encouraged, smiling, and challenged to respond to difficulties in the same spirit Miss Julia practices.

Meeting her in these pages and, even better, in person, you too will find help and comfort. Her faith and perseverance in Jesus Christ will urge you on through each day.

Sincerely,
Keith Lewis
Pastor, West Park Church of Christ,
Portsmouth, Virginia

I have come to know Julia Widlacki very well in the last couple of years since I have been her main home health nurse. Her courage in overcoming a life-changing event is awe-inspiring. Her sheer determination to walk after her accident is nothing short of a miracle. She is always upbeat and constantly has a smile on her face even though she is in constant pain. If I am having a bad day, she lifts me up with her upbeat ways. She praises God all the time and thanks him for everything she has come through. She is an amazing woman and has truly given her life over to God. I admire her strength, courage, and deep faith. Her book will be inspiring to everyone who reads it. It is an honor and a privilege to know this truly amazing woman and to call her my friend.

—Rose Marie King, RN

What an honor to have been asked to forward my comments in reference to Mother Julia's dynamic mission. I say mission because there are so many hurting families throughout the nations that need revelation and stabilization for life's ups and downs. Mother Julia has penned a beautiful book of her family autobiography to help others. Upon interviewing and reading her life story, the aroma of love comes from knowing her. The precious aroma doesn't match the pain and suffering that she has endured. Our Lord and Savior suffered to give us eternal life, and we must carry our cross. I have met none other like Mother Julia, who carries her cross daily.

Come with me and enjoy a trip over and through the rainbow of the mosaic colors of a book that was intricately inspired, *Rainbows After the Storms*. Through heartbreak, pain, tragedy, and of course, happiness and great gain, it is a beautiful family tapestry. It took great courage while convalescing from a tragic accident that had taken her mobility, to write her life story. It put me in remembrance of King David who penned the book of Psalms, and I'm sure we are going to hear more from her and her family in the near future.

—Silva Whitaker
Pastor of Shechaniah Rivers

Note to Readers: Pastor Whitaker was called to full time ministry in 1996 and has traveled as a missionary/evangelist to Africa. In 2006 she was ordained by Bishop T. D. Jakes and has planted over six churches. She is currently working as an evangelist planting Shechaniah Rivers' family services.

Jesus's love is pure!

07/16/2014

# Rainbows
## AFTER THE *Storms*

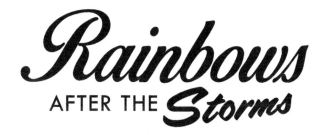

# Rainbows AFTER THE Storms

A
True Story
of a Quadraplegic
Mother and Her
Family
Overcoming
Tragedy

Julia Dean Childress Widlacki

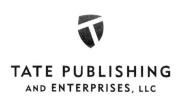

TATE PUBLISHING
AND ENTERPRISES, LLC

*Rainbows After the Storms*
Copyright © 2015 by Julia Dean Childress Widlacki. All rights reserved.

No part of this publication may be reproduced, stored in a retrieval system or transmitted in any way by any means, electronic, mechanical, photocopy, recording or otherwise without the prior permission of the author except as provided by USA copyright law.

Quoted Scriptures were taken from the *Saint Jerome's Catholic Study Bible*.

This book is designed to provide accurate and authoritative information with regard to the subject matter covered. This information is given with the understanding that neither the author nor Tate Publishing, LLC is engaged in rendering legal, professional advice. Since the details of your situation are fact dependent, you should additionally seek the services of a competent professional.

The opinions expressed by the author are not necessarily those of Tate Publishing, LLC.

Published by Tate Publishing & Enterprises, LLC
127 E. Trade Center Terrace | Mustang, Oklahoma 73064 USA
1.888.361.9473 | www.tatepublishing.com

Tate Publishing is committed to excellence in the publishing industry. The company reflects the philosophy established by the founders, based on Psalm 68:11,
"*The Lord gave the word and great was the company of those who published it.*"

Book design copyright © 2015 by Tate Publishing, LLC. All rights reserved.
*Cover design by Niño Carlo Suico*
*Interior design by Mary Jean Archival*

Published in the United States of America

ISBN: 978-1-63418-794-7
Biography & Autobiography / People with Disabilities
15.02.04

You gain strength, courage and confidence by every experience in which you really stop to look fear in the face. You are able to say to yourself, "I have lived through this horror. I can take the next thing that comes along." You must do the thing you think you cannot do.

—Eleanor Roosevelt, US Diplomat and Reformer (1884–1962)

# Dedication

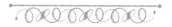

Above all, to my beloved Lord and Savior, Jesus Christ, for without him I would not be alive today.

To my wonderful children, their spouses, and my grandchildren, who have always been by my side encouraging and helping me in too many ways to mention. Without their love and support, I could not have gotten through the trials that I have faced over the years and that I still face today. I so deeply appreciate the love and constant care that Guy provides for me on a daily basis, as well as the ongoing love and support I receive from all of my children. I wish that I could do more to help each one of my children and grandchildren; it is my greatest wish that the Lord bless and care for them as much as he has me. I praise my Heavenly Father forever for his constant care and for all the help he has given me through my children.

Also, to my brothers and sisters who have always been supportive, especially my older brother, Clyde Childress, who, without his support, I could not have brought this book to fruition; to Carol Hummel for her wonderful support as my friend and ghostwriter, who has made my story come to life in this book. I cannot thank her enough.

She is a freelance writer, and her contact information is as follows:

20431 Payeras St.
Chatsworth, CA 91311
topnga1@aol.com
(818)590-4119

# Acknowledgments

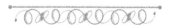

I want to thank my ex-husband, Don, for his hard work, support, and encouragement in the beginning and over the years. May God bless all of my friends and relatives who have always been there for me.

I also do not want to forget all of the wonderful pastors whom I have studied under, who have helped me grow in the ways of the Lord, and my wonderful pastor, Keith Lewis, of whom I now sit under with West Park Church of Christ in Portsmouth, Virginia; he is a wonderful man of God. I ask God's blessings on all of these pastors and pray they will all be end-time ministers.

I must not forget to thank Ross and Sharon Bagley. Sharon has been a constant source of help to me during the years that I have been living with my son, Guy. Sharon and Ross are lovely, caring people, and I pray that God will bless them abundantly.

I also wish to give special thanks to my beautiful daughter, Donna Hepner, for her help in compiling material, typing all my notes, and gathering pictures for this book. She has taken a great deal of her time to gather and review the materials and notes for this manuscript.

Each of my children has contributed a great deal of time and effort in the compilation of materials for my book, and I want to thank them sincerely for sharing their own unique perspectives on the events that affected our lives in the aftermath of my accident. I am eternally grateful for the love and help each of my children has unselfishly given me throughout these many years.

As my readers will discover, I was not the only one injured during my life-changing accident; some scars go deeper than the obvious physical ones.

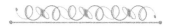

# Contents

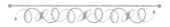

Introduction .................................................................. 19
The Event ..................................................................... 21
   Are You Trying to Kill Me? ..................................... 29
My Life before the Event .............................................. 31
Daddy, a Tortured Soul ................................................ 37
   Don Meets Daddy .................................................... 45
Young and Married ...................................................... 49
   The Difference .......................................................... 55
I Can and I Will…Walk ............................................... 57
   Don's Little Army .................................................... 59
   Coming Home…Almost .......................................... 65
   The Worst Trip Ever ................................................ 66
Home at Last ................................................................ 69
   Home from Vietnam, 1971 ...................................... 76
A Storm Strikes Again ................................................. 89
   Brother Clyde to the Rescue Again .......................... 91

More Than Enough! ............................................................... 97
   Until Death Do We Part…Again ...................................... 99
   More Surgeries ................................................................. 107

A Message from God .......................................................... 109
   The Lord Giveth (and Taketh Away) ............................... 110
   Medjugorje, Yugoslavia .................................................. 112
   My Easter Sunday Miracle .............................................. 113
   On Fire for the Lord ...................................................... 117
   A Peaceful Passing .......................................................... 120

A New Career? ................................................................... 123
   The Wedding Present ..................................................... 124
   The Letter I Never Sent .................................................. 125
   Life on My Own ............................................................ 130

Time for a Change ............................................................. 133
   Understanding God's Messages ...................................... 135
   Looking Back ................................................................. 136

My Loving Family: Their Stories ......................................... 137
   My Long-Suffering Grandmother ................................... 138
   Purpose .......................................................................... 140
   Mama ............................................................................. 141
   Reach for a Star ............................................................. 142
   They Were All Victims… ................................................ 145
   Sue Remembers ............................................................. 146
      Sue's Story (in Her Words) ....................................... 147
      The Hard Stuff… ...................................................... 149
   A New Beginning .......................................................... 153
   Donna's Story ................................................................ 155
   Tim's Worst Nightmare ................................................. 160
      Miracles happen ........................................................ 163

Donny's Long Struggle ............................................................. 165
   What Followed… ................................................................. 166
   Five-Year-Old Guy Heard the Crash ................................... 174

Don's View ................................................................................. 181
   The Interview with Dad by Donna Hepner ......................... 182
   The Accident (from Donna's Interview with Dad) ................ 186

And Now. .................................................................................. 191
   Living with My Youngest Son ............................................. 192
   My Vision ............................................................................. 195

Epilogue .................................................................................... 197

Don's Passing ............................................................................ 199

Appendix ................................................................................... 201

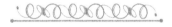

# Introduction

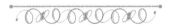

On a cold day in February 1967, the most devastating, life-shattering event happened that has changed my life, in every possible way, forever. It is my sincere hope that sharing my story will help and inspire others who may also be dealing with their own *mission impossible*.

The circumstances and specific details of your own personal derailment may be quite different from mine, but, believe me, I have stood in the most stark realization that nothing but God and my own indomitable spirit would carry me through the darkest days of my existence.

My prayer is that your own beautiful spirit will guide you through whatever trials you may be experiencing, and that it will lead you into the light. Our trials and battle wounds help make us warriors who, with the help of our loving God, will triumph over all adversity and be rewarded in *his* own time for our courage and valor.

My event happened over forty-seven years ago, but it remains as indelible today as though it happened yesterday. Had it not been for my faith in God and the positive attitude instilled in my spirit when I was only a child, I don't believe that I would have survived all that has happened to me.

It is not my intention to hurt or bring discredit upon anyone named in my book, but there are some difficult episodes and events that, should they be excluded, would not convey to my readers the impact that my accident had on everyone in my family, especially my beloved children, who have given me their permission to use their names and comments throughout these pages. Although the Lord has guided my steps through some extremely difficult times, the details of my struggle to survive must be told with complete integrity.

I hope that my emotional journey toward healing will encourage you, my readers, to believe in your own power and will to survive, and that you learn to rely on the Lord, who will surely hold each of you in the palm of his hand as he has me.

May God's greatest blessings be upon you.

—Julia Dean Childress Widlacki

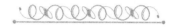

# The Event

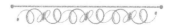

I was twenty-seven years old at the time, the mother of five young children, and happily married to Don Widlacki, a jet engine technician with the US Air Force.

The date was February 4, 1967, just another routine day as I drove home from the dentist's office with my eight-year-old son, Donny. We were laughing and chatting, just enjoying each other's company when, in my periphery, I saw bright lights where none should have been. I immediately realized that it was the headlights of another car coming head on toward us. Everything that followed seemed to have happened in a kind of surreal time warp. The terrible sounds of crashing metal, breaking glass, and the agonizing thud of my head hitting the windshield seemed to have happened in slow motion, but everything took place in a matter of seconds.

I knew I couldn't move my body and that I could hardly breathe, but the only thing running through my mind was my little boy, Donny. I called his name, over and over, but heard nothing except the indelible replay of shattering glass and crunching metal, and I knew that I was imprisoned in the wreckage of my car—a crushed and crushing cocoon of which a section had to be cut away in order to free me of its death grip on my body.

The next thing I remember was someone, a stranger, sitting in the passenger seat holding my head up so that I could get some air into my starving lungs. The kindness of this stranger perhaps saved my life as I would certainly have suffocated.

I heard the man say, "Ma'am, your son is okay," and I finally heard Donny's frightened little voice saying, "I'm okay, Mommy." Those words were the most precious my ears could have ever heard at that moment.

I knew I could deal with whatever happened to me, but I doubt that I could have ever lived through the loss of one of my children.

Immediately, I saw another bright light shining directly in my face, but this time it was a photographer from the *Wichita Eagle* newspaper who had jumped onto the hood of my car and taken a picture of us through the cracked windshield. By the time the photographer had snapped the picture, my husband, Don, had arrived and took over holding my head from the kind stranger. The picture below appeared in the *Wichita Eagle* newspaper the morning after my accident. When I was told about it, all I could think was, *What a way to get my picture in the newspaper!*

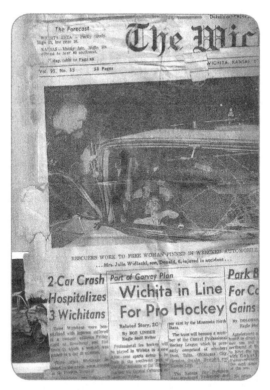

Newspaper clipping, *Wichita Eagle* February 4, 1967
*Outside left,* rescue worker; *inside left,* Donny
*Inside front,* me; *right,* Don, my husband

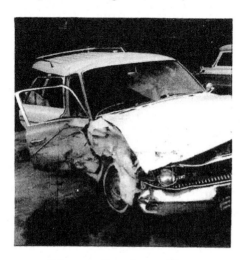

My car after the accident

My memories immediately after the crash have become somewhat fragmented. I recall only brief vignettes of the chaos that followed, but I do remember being taken by ambulance to the emergency room at the McDonald Military Hospital in Wichita, Kansas. I remember having the bloody clothes cut from my body and the persistent thought that *this could not be happening to me.*

It was quickly determined that the military hospital was not equipped to treat the devastating injuries I had sustained. Within an hour of my arrival, I had been transported to Wesley Medical Center, Wichita, Kansas, where the surgical team operated on my neck and placed tongs in my head attached to a forty-five-pound weight that held my neck stable and took the pressure off my spine. When I was finally able to see what had been done to me, it looked as though there was a giant ice pick sticking out from my head (the only method known in 1967) to secure my neck. When I awoke from surgery, I had no physical sensations from the neck down. I was lying in bed unable to move with the feeling that all of my internal organs were on fire.

The accident had broken my neck at the C5, C6, and C7 vertebrae; I was paralyzed from the neck down and classified as a quadriplegic—a medical term that conjures nightmare images of a dark and dire future for anyone who has or will ever receive that dreaded diagnosis.

My son, Donny, was kept at the military hospital for a few days because he had sustained a head concussion and some bruises. I had difficulty believing anyone who told me that Donny was fine since I was not able to see my children for two or three months after the accident. I suspected that no one wanted to tell me the truth about Donny's condition because of what I had been through, but on Easter Sunday, the hospital staff made it possible for me to speak to my children through some type of video intercom. I was finally able to see that Donny was truly okay, and I thank the Lord every day that he survived without lasting *physical* injuries (more on that later).

One of the nurses came in to check on me and asked, "So, how are *we* doing today?"

I was thinking, *I don't know about you, but I am in terrible pain. I'm sick and feel as though I am on fire, and I'm very frightened!*

"How can I help you, sweetie?" the nurse said with kindness. I asked for pain medication, and she told me that I had already been given some, but she would increase the dosage if I needed it. I was grateful for her concern and thanked her. She then asked, "Do you know where you are?" I told her that my head hurt very badly and that I could not move my body. She said, very soothingly, "Just try to relax. You have suffered severe injury, and the pain is probably from the tongs we have placed in your head." She told me that the doctor would be in to see me and answer all of my questions.

Soon the doctor was standing over me, explaining that I had broken my neck and that it would take some time to see how things would go. He said that they would do everything possible to make me comfortable, and if I had more questions, he would try to answer them. He gave me a sympathetic smile and said that my husband was waiting to see me.

I was still in shock but so grateful that Don was there. When he came into the room and saw me hooked up and wired up, he looked very frightened. I'm sure he tried his best to hide his fears from me by saying some humorous things to cheer me up, but I had to tell him to stop because my body hurt too much when I laughed.

With all of the newly added responsibilities for Don at home, I knew how hard this was for him. The Air Force allowed him some off-duty time for a while and provided some Red Cross services to assist him with the care of the children while I lay in the intensive care unit of the hospital for fifteen days, unable to make a single voluntary move.

During those first days after the accident, I was often in unbearable pain, but I tried to keep a positive attitude, asking always for the Lord's help. The staff would work my arms and legs as I lay in bed, and once, they placed a pillow on my chest that felt like a cinderblock. Even with so little weight barely pressing on my chest, I could hardly breathe, so they quickly removed it.

With only my brain in motion, all of my waking thoughts were spent on a single directive to my brain: "Move my big toe!" I literally pushed my brain to cooperate.

On the fifteenth day, my toe actually *moved*! One of the nurses noticed it and yelled aloud, "Her big toe moved!" Everyone in ICU began rejoicing for me. Someone immediately called the doctor to come and see my great accomplishment.

After that small milestone, I was finally taken out of ICU and placed in the special care unit where I was placed in a circle bed where I stayed for the next four months. The circle bed was the first one ever used by the hospital, and I was their guinea pig since most people at that time were put in a Stryker frame bed that turned the patient from side to side with jerky movements.

The circle bed, however, provided a much smoother transition as it rotated. Daily, I would be rotated from two hours lying on my back to two hours on my stomach, which helped keep my body from forming bed sores—a condition that almost always occurs in bedridden patients.

During the many hours that I spent lying on my stomach in the circle bed, I was provided with a pair of prism glasses that enabled me to see backward (over my shoulder) so that I could watch television. This helped me pass those interminably long hours with something besides my restless mind to keep me from becoming too depressed.

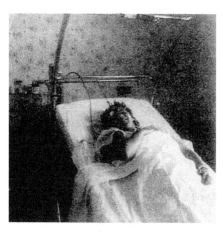
Me in the hospital's first circle bed.

I continued to force my mental energy toward other parts of my body, and soon I was able to move my arms, though not my hands.

Don was at the hospital every day, twice a day, to feed me. I can't even imagine how stressful this was for him with the five children at home to tend as well as his demanding job at the Air Force base. As difficult as all of this was for me to endure, I was heartsick for Don, who now had too much extra work and pressure—all of it because of me. It didn't matter that none of this was my fault; I still felt guilty about the extra burdens that Don had to bear alone.

As day after each long day passed, I wondered why all of this was happening to me. I prayed to God for his mercy and for the strength to endure my suffering. I asked his forgiveness for any wrong I might have done against him or for any hurt I might have caused others. I prayed that he would allow his love to shine through me so that I might help others even in the weakened state that I now found myself.

When Don came to visit, it was the high point of each day, and he always seemed to know the right things to say, but he couldn't successfully hide the sadness and concern in his eyes. This made me more determined than ever; I had to get up and walk, no matter how long it took. I wanted and needed my life back.

In the months ahead, I had vivid images while I was awake and asleep—images of all the things I would do when I could walk again.

Oh, yes, I never for a moment thought I would never walk again. I'm sure this stubbornness upset my caretakers and my husband to hear me insist on doing something that none of them believed was possible, given my dire condition.

I am not saying that I never felt discouraged, but when I did, I would quickly think of something positive that would help me get through those dark moments. I hardly ever gave into tears, but on one occasion, I felt so sad when Don left after a nice visit that I broke down and cried. It was during one of these moments when a doctor whom I had never seen before happened to pass by my room. He came inside and stood for a moment watching me before saying something in a none too friendly tone, "What do you have to cry about? There are so many people worse off than you are." Then before leaving my room, he looked back and added, "Snap out of it. Get yourself together and be glad that you're alive." I was stunned! This man didn't know me—knew nothing about me nor what I had been through—and he wasn't even my doctor. He probably had the idea that I was lying there feeling sorry for myself, but I rarely gave into thoughts like that. I was just lonely for my family.

Maybe the doctor was trying to use reverse psychology on me, or maybe he had lost someone close to him that had caused him to say such hurtful remarks. I do know that it was the wrong way to handle the situation, but I hold no hard feelings toward him. Instead, he taught me a valuable lesson through that painful experience.

I learned not to judge other people because it's difficult for any of us to know the depth of another's burdens or pains. Onlookers can't understand the degree of hardship or suffering another person has endured, and most of us have some form of buried wounds and sorrows that we don't allow others to see.

## Are You Trying to Kill Me?

A new nurse came to rotate the circle bed from the faceup to facedown position, but she had not screwed the top on tightly enough to rotate the bed safely. As the bed began to turn, I had a sense of falling followed by the lights going out and the electrical cord from the bed sending sparks through the hospital room. Apparently, the cord had gotten twisted around the wheel of the bed and had torn in half. There was a great deal of panic and commotion as the attendants tried to lower me from a forty-five-degree angle to facedown. I wasn't used to being suspended at that angle, and the pressure made me pass out. I was deathly afraid that the tongs holding my head stable would be pulled out during the chaos. I called out, "I think you all are trying to kill me!"

The nurses continued wiping my face with wet cloths to keep me calm. Finally, someone used the manual crank to turn the bed to the down position, and I had to stay that way until the electrician came and fixed all of the electrical problems.

When Don came to visit and heard what had happened, he was so angry that he demanded no one be permitted to touch the bed or handle any portion of my care who didn't know what they were doing.

I had many trials and setbacks during the eight months I was hospitalized at Wesley Medical Center, but one of the hardest for me, or for anyone who was raised with the modesty common to young women of my time, was the loss of privacy. This became a daily reminder of my complete dependency. Each time a nurse or hospital attendant had to change my soiled clothing, wash my body, or wipe my nose, I felt more and more helpless and humiliated. Of course, I appreciated those who were willing to do such things for me, but there is no greater loss of dignity than to lose control over one's private functions. I wish I could say that I eventually got used to it, but I truly never did.

Part of my routine care was the ritual of cleaning my nose. The nurses used a suction device, much like the rubber squeeze ball used on a baby's nose when he or she is unable to blow by themselves. One of the nurses charged with this duty was so rough during the procedure that I dreaded seeing her enter my room. Her manner was so harsh, in fact, that she often brought tears of pain to my eyes.

I didn't have the nerve to complain because I was at the mercy of anyone administering every type of care for me. The word "helpless" (for me) had grown in scope from a rather innocuous word to something the size of a mountain by comparison.

Part of my therapy was geared to increasing my lung capacity. When patients are bedridden, they tend to breathe in a more shallow manner than when they are mobile, and this often becomes a catalyst for hospital-related pneumonia.

One day, when I had the breathing mask over my face, the therapist was engaged in a lively conversation with one of my family members and wasn't paying close enough attention to me. When my breathing therapy session was over and it was time to remove the mask, the therapist was still distracted and didn't notice that I was in distress. I began moaning, but the breathing machine was too loud for my muffled sounds to be heard. When the therapist finally looked at me, he realized that I was about to blow up! He ran to me in a state of panic and couldn't apologize enough for his negligence.

As you can see, there were many ways for me to die in the hospital, even while being treated in the *special care unit*.

# My Life before the Event

I was born the second oldest of six children into a family where a great deal of emotional and physical abuse was the rule rather than the exception. I believe that because of the trials I endured in childhood, I was better able to handle the "trials" and ordeals that happened to me in the hospital and thereafter.

I gained spiritual strength from an early age because I learned from my mother to look to the Lord as the only true source of peace, trust, and security, which were lacking in our home.

I was blessed to have an older brother, Clyde, just two years older than I, who always looked after me and became my closest friend and confidant during childhood and throughout our adolescent years. We have remained exceptionally close even after we each left home to find our own life's journeys.

Clyde has published his own remarkable autobiography, *Forks: The Life of One Marine*, which recounts, in part, what life was like for him during our post-WWII childhood, especially as it pertains to his relationship with our father.

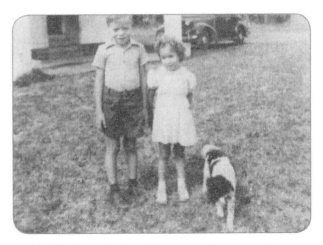

My big brother Clyde, me, and our dog Spot

I grew up in the country and loved the outdoors, the smell of the fresh air, and the wide-open spaces that allowed me to run fast and free, and to enjoy the beauty of the world around me. Appropriately, my favorite song was "Don't Fence Me In."

I loved exploring the forest, finding buried treasure, watching the abundant wildlife (that I always tried to catch). I also developed a very special love for animals—a love that has never diminished over the years. I have always felt that animals were my friends, and I believed that I could always love and trust them more than I could trust people. Later on, my husband would find out just how much I loved animals when he had to build pens and cages for my ever-growing menagerie.

As I have already alluded, my family was not *normal* by any traditional definition, but my mother tried her best to be a stabilizing influence—the teacher and nurturer for us all. She was the one who single-handedly kept our family together. She was a true Christian, and everything we learned about love and compassion came from her words and example. I know that my developing spirit was fed solely by her, and it has given me the ability to survive many of life's difficulties. I saw how much emotional suffering my mother endured, and she did it with astounding humility and grace.

Suffering changes people; it can either harden a person's heart or soften it, and I'm grateful that my mother's loving demeanor never changed despite how justified she would have been to turn the other way.

I remember the times when I would sit on our outdoor swing just talking to God. I learned that talking directly to him always gave me a feeling of peace. I absolutely believed that he was listening and that he loved me.

My father's spiritual nature (or lack thereof) was a totally different story. Although he proclaimed to believe in God, the Creator, and said that he "talked to him every night," my father did not believe in Jesus Christ, therefore, proclaimed himself an agnostic.

My father also had a split personality, much like the famed *Dr. Jekyll and Mr. Hyde*. In one moment, he could be so cruel that I hated him, and in another, he could be so nice that I couldn't help loving him. The problem was that we never knew what would trigger the appearance of the dreaded "Mr. Hyde."

I believe it was because of my father's cruelty and my need for spiritual and emotional security that I came to the Lord early in life, about the age of seven. I even thought that I would like to become a nun, although we weren't Catholic.

I have already mentioned that without warning, my father would suddenly be overcome with extreme anger, and I will never forget some of those occasions. One night, while I was sleeping, he came home from our family-owned drive-in theater and jerked me out of bed and proceeded to beat me, as always, with the buckle end of his belt until blood was pouring down my legs and I could not even stand up. Why he did this, I will never know, but things like that happened frequently, and when our mother tried to stop him from whipping us, he would turn and start beating on her as well.

My older brother, Clyde, with all of his young outrage, often tried to stop him, but my father was especially hard on Clyde. I felt very sorry for my brother and tried to console him after some of my father's raging episodes that were directed toward him.

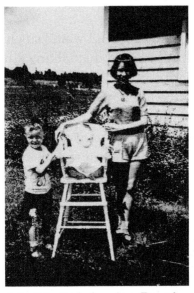

Left to right My little brother, David, my sister, Connie, in the highchair, and me

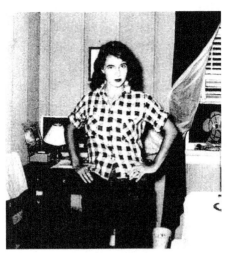

Me at age 14

One time Clyde told me that he planned to run away from home, and I remember begging him to take me with him. Clyde actually did manage to sneak away and purchased a bus ticket to the home where one of our relatives lived. Unfortunately, my father had called the police and alerted them to where Clyde might be headed. He further instructed the police that when they found him, they were to put Clyde in jail until my father could come to get him.

When my father was upset about something, it was his custom to sit at the kitchen table with whomever he deemed responsible for his displeasure and engage the "culprit" in one of his interminable lectures. I remember one time when I had gotten a bad grade on a math test, and he made me sit down on the kitchen stool all night while he yelled and lectured me. When I would inevitably begin to fall asleep, he would start hitting me.

I and all of my brothers and sisters went through a lot, but our mother was treated just as badly, if not worse. Clyde and I were the oldest, and though we were small, we often tried to stick up for each other and for our mother.

I recall shaking in my shoes, begging him to "Leave my momma alone!." He yelled back at me, saying, "Get away, or I will knock your teeth down your throat!"

For spiritual guidance, my brother and I went to a local Baptist church where I was baptized at the age of twelve. After attending that church for about a year, I felt that the people in the congregation were hypocrites because they were always gossiping. I had overheard many of their judgmental remarks about other church members, even criticisms about the clothes that some of the members wore to church. There were also a number of people in the congregation who didn't like the way the preacher delivered his sermons, so they forced him to leave. I was sad to see this happen, so I left the church never to return. It wasn't until after I married my husband, who was Catholic, that I also joined the Catholic church so that we might raise our children in the same faith and worship together as a family. I finally felt that I had found my spiritual home because no one seemed to sit in judgment of their fellow parishioners.

Was it hard to forgive my father? Yes, it was, but later on I knew that if I did not forgive him, I would also not be forgiven for my own sins. I knew this because the Lord had instilled in me that spiritual insight. I tried always to follow in the Lord's ways even though I sometimes felt as though I was a sinner not worthy of his love.

# Daddy, a Tortured Soul

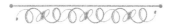

My father truly was a tortured soul. He was a man with a raging, conflicted personality. I can remember a time when, in his own words, he admitted that he was "a woman in a man's body."

Daddy eventually sought a sex change operation after reading the publicity about Christine Jorgenson's successful sex reassignment surgery that took place in Denmark in 1952. The former GI named George Jorgensen became the focus of worldwide attention when he opted to undergo the radical surgery to become a woman, and later, *she* was credited as the "pioneer of the sexual revolution."

Personally encouraged by all the new research in sex reassignment surgery, my father drove our family to Johns Hopkins Hospital in Baltimore, Maryland, so that he could be interviewed for a possible sex change.

Clyde and I were also interviewed during our father's application process, and I believe he may have been denied the operation because of the things that Clyde and I revealed about his emotional instability. I feel certain that there must have been some concerns about how the sex change might have affected him, but more particularly, how it might have affected his wife and children.

Certain things became worse after my father was denied the sex change operation. At home, he began dressing in women's clothes, wearing wigs and makeup, and causing all of us to feel extremely uncomfortable.

Of course, we were all too embarrassed to invite friends to visit for fear they would see our father and begin to ask a lot of humiliating questions. Sometimes he would even make our mother dress as a man.

As afraid of our father as we children were, our mother was terrified of him and always did what she was told or would suffer the consequences. Ironically, when father dressed as a woman, he was much kinder, but when dressed as a man, he was cruel and often violent.

Surprisingly, Mother continued to have children. My brother, David, was born ten years after Clyde and I, followed by my sister, Connie, then, quite a bit later, a set of twins, Gary and Sherry. It was difficult to bond with the younger children because by the time they were born, I was married and living out of state with a family of my own.

I often wondered how Mother endured the chaos and erratic behavior of our father, but somehow she continued to bear it all with uncommon grace. There were times when I witnessed my father sitting alone in the living room with tears in his eyes, and I wished that I could just have an honest conversation with him about his feelings. You might imagine how it must have been for someone like him back in the 1950s when the idea of sexual identity was never mentioned, at least not in any public forum that we knew of.

When I was quite young, my father molested me for a few years. I felt terribly ashamed and finally got up the courage to tell my mother. She talked to him about it, but like the rest of us, she had little power or influence over him. She found herself in the same position as many women of that time—with no place to go, no real job skills, and no education. She continued to live with him in order to take care of her children. Eventually the abuse stopped.

There were times when I tried to talk to my father when I wanted to help him accept the Lord as his Savior, which I believe he may have before he died.

Daddy gave me my first horse, a pinto that I named Beauty. Whether he gave me the horse out of guilt or love, I still do not know, but caring for Beauty taught me a lot about taking responsibility for another living thing and how to care for animals in general. But with all of the wonderful memories I have of my first horse, he often scared me by running away with me on his back. He was so big that I could hardly control him, and it was only by the grace of God that I was not killed while riding him. One day when he ran away with me, I just knew that God was protecting me when I wasn't thrown off and killed before he finally came to a stop at the edge of a road.

Another close call was the time when Beauty took off down the main highway and turned ninety degrees at a farm so that he could see the other horses; I was barely able to hold on. Had I been thrown off, I might not have missed the barbed wire fence. During those occasions, I often felt that the Lord must have had other plans for me, or I would surely not have survived.

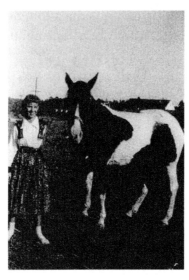

Me and my first horse 'Beauty'

Following my father's sexual, mental, and other types of physical abuses against me, I found it difficult to forget all that he had done to me and to the rest of my family. Later on, after the sexual abuse stopped, he never talked about the things that he had done, but I felt certain they must have haunted him because of the dark, reflective moods that I often witnessed. My father was possibly an enigma even to himself.

I know that his cross-dressing put its mark on all of us, as well as on our mother, but I believe we all came to forgive him and tried to keep the past where it belonged.

Father used to say, "Walk a mile in my shoes before judging me." It was a lesson that I learned early and one that has been reinforced many times over the years as I have matured. Father had his demons to fight, and I understood some of his pain while fighting my own. We learn, grow, and mature through our own trials, and our character is determined by how we weather those trials.

I would not be entirely fair if I didn't also mention the better side of my father. He was a self-made man, an entrepreneur, and a man of exceptionally high intelligence. He and my brother

Clyde built a twelve-foot reflector telescope in our backyard that was visited by many people who, after talking to both of them, believed they were professional astronomers (Clyde was just a teenager at the time).

Because of my father's entrepreneurial spirit, he built the first drive-in movie theater in the state of Virginia. As a family, we ran a thriving business that kept all of us working long hours, seven days a week, often late into the night. But working hard also meant that I earned my own money and had the freedom to use my earnings for whatever I wished.

When I was sixteen years old, I had saved enough money to buy my second horse, a palomino that I named Tarzan.

My father was surprisingly supportive and even built a barn and corral for Tarzan.

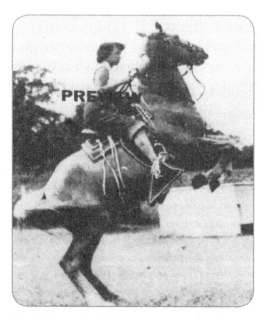

Tricks I taught Tarzan—photo courtesy of *Richmond Times-Dispatch*

When I first bought Tarzan, I had to nurture him back to health because the previous owners had not taken good care of him. I trained him to do all kinds of tricks: to nod for "yes," to move his head from side to side for "no," and to raise his leg to simulate shaking hands. Eventually, I taught him how to jump. I rode him in the Tobacco Festival in Richmond, Virginia, one year and showed his tricks off at several different horse shows.

I used to ride him to school quite a lot during the school year because the other kids enjoyed seeing him do the tricks I had taught him.

On one occasion, when I was riding Tarzan in the woods, we came across a huge gully, so I had to get him to jump over it. When he jumped, I fell off, and his left front hoof landed on my arm just inches from my head. During the times that I owned my two horses, I experienced several accidents, but I loved my horses and never considered that my hobby might be too dangerous for me. I later had to sell Tarzan because I had gotten married and we were restationed with Don's air force career to a base in Texas. I just knew that horse training was a career that I was well suited because after giving Tarzan my tender loving care, someone offered to buy him for five hundred dollars—ten times the amount I had paid for him.

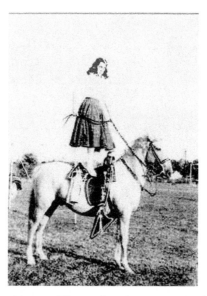

Me standing on Tarzan/performing with Tarzan'

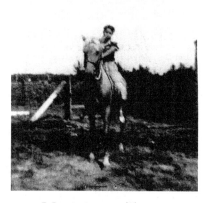

Me sitting on Tarzan

Along with training wild horses, I had begun performing interpretive dance, a passion that turned from a hobby into the beginning of a serious profession.

My brother Clyde had always loved listening to classical music, another influence we both enjoyed from our mother. Clyde studied French horn in high school and played in the all-state high school band competition. At home, when Clyde played classical music recordings, I could feel the music moving through me, and I would always dance along, making up my own dance routines. By classification, I was an interpretive dancer. The music that flowed through my body dictated the story I portrayed through my movements. I loved all kinds of music and felt that I had been given a natural, God-given talent for expressing myself through dance.

At fifteen years old, I won a talent contest that was sponsored by a local television station. After I had won, the station paid me to perform live, once a week, on a show called *Teenage Dance Party*.

My dreams of becoming a dance professional were always in the forefront of my mind. I even thought it might be possible for me to become a dancer in musicals, which were very big film genres at that time.

I had also begun taking flying lessons after my brother Clyde, at seventeen years old, became the youngest licensed pilot in the state of Virginia. I actually have eight hours of flying time, but over the years, I have misplaced my logbook.

My very active young life before the age of eighteen was filled with dancing, horse training, and flying lessons; all of which came crashing down eleven years later. Had I known what was in store for me, I don't think I could have survived the shock.

I doubt there is a single human being who expects their life to change as dramatically as mine did, but these things happen all the time. At the age of twenty-seven years, I went from a life filled with possibilities of becoming all I had dreamed to a life that quickly became just a memory.

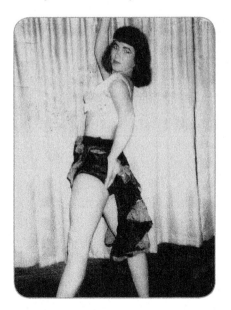

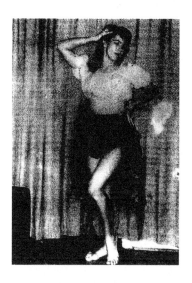

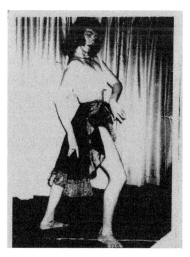

Dancing made me feel free—I believed that I was born to dance.

## Don Meets Daddy

I first met my husband, Don, along with a buddy of his at the local skating rink on the night before Easter Sunday, 1956.

When my brother Clyde came to pick me up afterward, he had a chance to meet Don, and he told me that he "approved."

My big brother's approval was not a thing casually given. Clyde had always scrutinized the character of other guys who showed interest in me, and he often warned me about someone with whom he thought I should not associate.

The next day, on Easter Sunday, Don came to our house to meet my parents. A week later, Don came to see me again, late at night and unannounced. When the car came roaring up our driveway, my father (thinking we had an intruder) took a gun that he kept in the house and went out the front door. He fired the gun in the air and told Don to get out of the car. Don's buddies acted as though they were scared to death and drove off as fast as they could go, leaving Don standing there to face my father—alone.

My father started fussing at Don and scared him half to death. The scene was like something out of the movies when a father takes out his shotgun and threatens to shoot the amorous boyfriend.

I wondered what was going to happen next, and I'll bet Don was thinking of every way imaginable to escape the scene without getting shot.

I never actually knew the reason for his odd behavior, but perhaps my father enjoyed having some fun at Don's expense because shortly after that very threatening scene, he invited Don into the house. I thought it was brave of Don to stay, but I guess he liked me a lot or didn't want to appear a coward, so he accepted my father's invitation.

Now my father liked to talk, so he continued to lecture Don long after they went inside; and when my father started talking, a person might as well get ready for an all-nighter.

Imagine being confronted by an angry father with a gun who, by the way, was dressed as a woman the night that Don met him. I kept looking at Don out of the corner of my eye for his reaction, but he sat there listening to my father, thinking, I'm sure, *What in the world have I gotten myself into!*

Remarkably, Don didn't judge my father. After patiently listening to him prattle on about something for quite a while, my father actually invited Don to spend the night since we lived in the country, and it was a long way back to the naval base, where he was stationed. Don had also been drinking that night. I don't know if my father knew that he was carrying a flask in his pants pocket, but I expect had he known, Don would have been in store for another lengthy lecture and perhaps a boot out the door.

I didn't drink and vowed that I would never start after witnessing the terrible things that happened due to my grandfather's alcoholism and how it affected his whole life and family. I told myself that I would never marry anyone who drank, but Don and I loved each other, and it just goes to show that you can never say never and actually know whether you can keep that kind of promise.

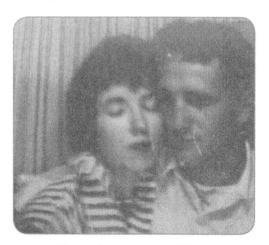

Young love—me and Don

Don and I became engaged in August and decided to get married in December, less than a year after we met, because Don was getting ready to ship out for a long deployment, and we wanted to get married before he left.

Oddly, my father and Don grew to have a great relationship, and in some good ways, they were quite a bit alike.

# Young and Married

There we were, married! A country girl and a city boy, but we made it work—at least for the next thirty-three years. When we first fell in love, I was convinced that Don and I were a perfect match, and I believed he liked many of the same things that I did. He was a wonderful man, but I found out, once the rose-colored glasses lost some of their tint, we had many divergent tastes and viewpoints.

For one thing, Don was jealous of my dancing, and for another, he didn't like animals—both extremely important to me.

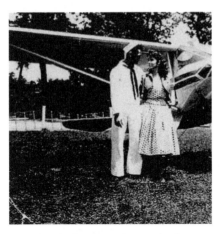

Don and me in the early days

Don continued to feel extremely jealous of my dancing after we were married, but I loved to dance and believed that all talents are gifts from God.

I wanted to be a good wife as much as I believed God wanted me to be. When I danced, I felt that I danced for him. After a while, I began questioning my desire to dance in view of my husband's jealousy and started thinking that I might be putting my own desires above those of God, and in so doing, I was engaged in something that did not honor my husband.

This realization came to me when I stopped caring that Don was jealous of my dancing because it gave me such pleasure.

Don told me that he did not like to watch me dance in public because I was not dancing for him but for other people. On those occasions when I tried to dance for Don at home, he would always want me to go to bed with him, which often made me feel cheap and dirty because it reminded me of being sexually molested as a child. For me, dancing was something pure that allowed me to become engrossed in the joy of feeling the music. Looking back on these memories, I pray that my ex-husband will forgive me for this, since it clearly put a strain on our marriage. I hope that one day he would be able to understand the complexity of my mixed emotions about this sensitive issue.

I eventually asked the Lord to bring me back to him and to forgive me for straying off the path.

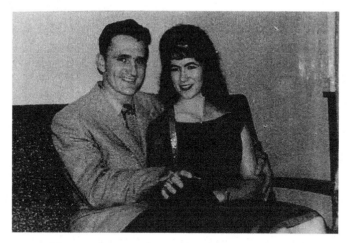

Don and me in Japan during happier days

Our first child, Donna, was born nine months after we got married, and because Don was often out to sea, we lived with my parents during this time. When he returned home from one of his missions, Don had to make a decision about staying in the Navy or changing military affiliations because with the Navy, he was gone from home much too often. This was a very difficult decision for Don because he had loved being in the Navy. After much deliberation, he decided to join the Air Force so that he could be at home with his family more often. But, by making this change, Don lost two stripes in rank, and he was required to make a change in career fields.

We left for Wichita Falls, Texas, for Don's training as a jet engine technician—the new career field he had chosen because he was told that it was a wide-open field with many future opportunities for advancement. This, however, was not the case. Once Don graduated from school, he found out that his career choice had been frozen for seven years, which meant that he could not progress in rank during that time. You can imagine how difficult it was for us to raise our five young children on an airman third class' pay; it was not until Don was stationed in Japan that he received a raise in rank from airman third class to staff sergeant.

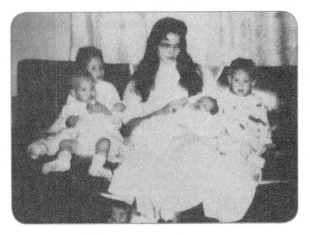

Me and my growing family

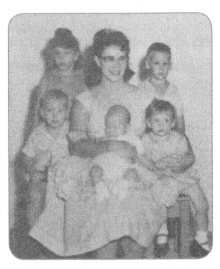

*Back row,* Donna, me, and Donny; *front row,* Tim, Guy, and Susie

When we returned to the United States, we were stationed in Wichita, Kansas, which was where my accident occurred that adversely affected our entire family in one way or another from that time forward.

I would be lying if I didn't admit that because of the events that stole my once extremely athletic youth, I often felt abandoned—abandoned by my husband, my true love, whom, over the course of our thirty-three-year marriage, I had never stopped loving.

Through all of our difficulties, Don was a model of strength, courage, and perseverance. He did more for me during those early days after the accident than I can name, but what happened between us rocked the very foundation of the lives we had both dreamed of as individuals and as a couple. I cannot blame my husband because he did everything he could do to help, but in the final analysis, he also had to address his own needs. I continue to feel very sad for Don having lost his own dreams and for being forced to make decisions that ultimately caused him pain regardless of his choices.

Despite wanting to be objective, most people understand that there is more than one side to any story. Don and I were a young married couple with an emotional investment in our marriage and in the lives of our children, but we were individually responsible for our own happiness.

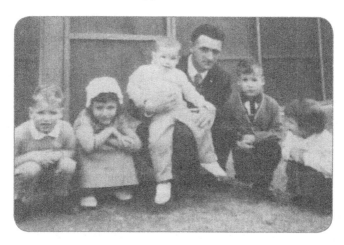

*Left to right:* Tim, Donna, Guy, Don, Donny, and Susie

After the accident, all I could think about besides learning to walk again was how I was going to be a good wife to my husband and a good mother to my children. I pleaded with God, asking him for his blessing that would allow me to walk again. I dreamed of walking out of the hospital on my own two feet, but I knew that I could only do this through the grace and mercy of the Lord. I prayed constantly for his blessings that would help me not become a constant burden to my husband and children.

I rededicated my life back to the Lord. Since that time, I have tried to put him first in everything I think, say, and do.

I often reflect on times past, but mostly, I wonder what lay ahead. As you read on, you will see that much has happened to the country girl with the big dreams of becoming a professional horse trainer and dancer.

Dreams keep us striving to become all that we can be in this (relatively speaking) short lifetime, but fate often intervenes, and our dreams become like dandelion fluff in the wind. When something unexpected happens that changes everything, we are forced to recalibrate our lives, start over, and to create an entirely different life plan.

Today I choose to think only of the good things from my childhood: My mother, my brothers and sisters, the family trips to the mountains, and camping. We had our share of those things too, and only once in a while, I remember the dark clouds that pass briefly over my memories. I choose to see the sunshine in the clear blue sky at day and the bright moon- and star-filled sky at night—beautiful reminders that life, with all of its hardships, is still worth living and loving if we allow ourselves to overcome the obstacles. I would like to share the following poem with you—a perfect reminder of how we gain strength each day by invoking God's help, no matter what we may encounter.

## The Difference

I got up early one morning,
And rushed right into the day;
I had so much to accomplish
That I didn't take time to pray.

Problems just tumbled about me,
And heavier came each task,
"Why doesn't God help me?" I wondered
He answered, "You didn't ask."

I wanted to see joy and beauty,
But the day toiled on, gray and bleak
I wondered why God didn't show me,
He said, "But you didn't seek."

I tried to come into God's presence,
I used all my keys at the lock;
God gently and lovingly chided,
"My child, you didn't knock."

I woke up early this morning,
And paused before entering the day;
I had so much to accomplish
That I had to take time to pray.

—Anonymous

# I Can and I Will...Walk

I hadn't seen my children during the first four months that I remained hospitalized in Wichita, Kansas, because I was confined to the circle bed, and children were not permitted to visit. After the four-month mark, the doctors removed the tongs from my head and placed a steel neck brace around my neck that rested on my shoulders to stabilize my head.

It was now time for me to begin rehabilitation therapy sessions. I was transported, by wheelchair, to the therapy room, but I often passed out because I had been lying in bed for so long that the added pressure on the nerves in my spine caused me to lose consciousness. During these therapy sessions, I was placed on a tilt table that was designed to help bedridden patients transition from lying in bed for weeks or months to sitting upright in a wheelchair. The therapists would strap me to the table and gradually raise the head of the table a little higher each time. I did this exercise every day until it became easier for me to remain upright for longer periods of time without passing out. My therapy sessions also consisted of exercising my hands, arms, and legs. These were not easy workouts for me, and by the time I was taken back to my bed, I was exhausted. Although I still could not use my hands and had no feeling from my chest down, I became gradually stronger and more encouraged each day.

Finally, the day came when I could sit upright in a wheelchair, and Don was permitted to wheel me into the hospital visitor's room where I could visit with my children. We were elated to see each other! I think the children thought I would break because they gingerly placed their arms around me and gave me gentle hugs and kisses. Don had prepared the children for our visit, but I could see their anxious little faces and knew they must have a thousand questions they needed answered about me and what the future held for all of us.

I can't begin to express how wonderful this was. Don had kept me up-to-date on the children's activities, but as nice as that was to hear about their day-to-day activities, it was no substitute for seeing their beautiful faces. I thanked God that I could still do that.

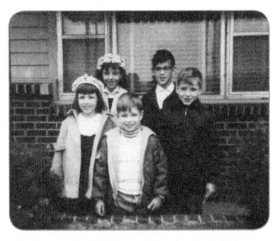

*Left to right: Back row,* Donna and Donny; *middle row,* Susie and Tim; *front row,* Guy

## Don's Little Army

Don told me that our neighbors brought home-cooked meals for him and the children, and they helped in other ways, but those things tapered off after a while. My mother came to stay with us for about a month until my father wanted her home, so the pressure of taking exclusive care of our home and children was back on his shoulders.

Don's military commander was great, as was the entire base. Don said his supervisors allowed him enough time at home in the morning until the last child got to school before reporting for work and would allow him to leave early in order to be home when all of the children returned. The school allowed Guy (the youngest) to stay after school until everyone else was ready to go home so that he wouldn't be left alone. Don was also permitted time off to feed me lunch at the hospital, and he later confessed that he was probably away from work more than he was there. Everyone who knew about my accident tried to be of as much help as they could be. Don's superior officers and the base, in general, gave him enough relief so that he could still work and not lose his job when he was unable to be there.

The children remember the things they did for fun as a family while I was in the hospital that consisted of trips to the park, playing in the yard, and watching TV (after chores were done). On the weekends, Don would come to the hospital to help feed me breakfast while the children had been trained to take care of chores around the house and look out after each other while he was gone. Don taught the children that if they worked together, I could come home sooner. He said that the children gave him no problems as they all wanted to see me again and kept asking about me, whether I was going to be okay and when they could see me again. He said that the children were like his little army, and he ran the house like a general. He said he would have been put in child protective services if he did the same today, but he kept the family together, and they always did everything together.

I was extremely restricted in my movements, but I felt a small degree of freedom when I, at last, felt another milestone had been reached in my recovery. Because I had begun to show steady progress, I was moved from the special care unit to a regular hospital room where I also gained a roommate.

Each day they would weigh me and place a pair of snug tights on my legs that were supposed to aid in my circulation. Believe me, getting into those things was a struggle that I never looked forward to. I felt like a sausage too big for its casing. The process was grueling! The staff member helping me would slide me from my wheelchair onto the scales to weigh me, and it was so awkward that I began asking them to let me stand on the scales by myself. I was absolutely positive that I could do it; my brain said so, and I believed my brain.

In the therapy room, in front of the tilt table, there was a set of parallel bars that I thought looked sturdy enough for me to hold onto. I felt I could use the strength of my upper arms and rest my weight on them in order to take a few steps. I believe the therapy staff grew so tired of my insistence that they finally gave in, unstrapped me, and let me try.

As I reached for the parallel bars directly in front of me, my arms were weaker than a baby's, and I collapsed onto the floor on the first try. The therapists picked me up off the floor, placed me on a gurney, and took me back to my room and put me to bed. You might think this would deter me from thinking I would walk one day, but my determination only grew stronger. I kept telling my brain, "I can walk. I can do this!"

After quite a few therapy sessions (and a great deal of begging on my part), the attendants unstrapped me once again with, I expect, a few eye-rolling exchanges between them. They had to be growing weary of my constant, *unrealistic* insistence that I could walk, and so humor me they did. But, this time, I did it! I took one step and passed out over the therapist's shoulder and woke up in my hospital bed. This was the moment I had been working for, the milestone that would change everything. By taking the first daring step, I knew that my goal to walk again was drawing closer each day. I was thrilled; my therapists were thrilled. Although I had no feeling in my legs, I had somehow gotten my legs to move.

I continued daily therapy sessions on the tilt table for quite some time. I also began using a variety of exercise machines and equipment to help my muscles grow stronger. I was also put in a whirlpool tub every day to further revive my sluggish circulation. Slowly, I was able to walk a few steps using a four-legged walker.

Throughout the long days, weeks, and months when I wasn't consumed with all of the physically demanding recuperative therapies, I worked hard on my ongoing emotional struggle to forgive my father for the terrible things that I and my family had endured at his hands. I found the best way to do this was to remember the good things that he had also done for us.

Once when my parents made the trip from Virginia to visit me in the hospital, my father sat in the chair beside my bed and did his best to cheer me up—a talent he had but didn't often use.

He squeezed my hand and said, "You *will* walk. Remember the story of *The Little Engine that Could*? The Little Engine That Could was trying to chug up a very difficult hill and kept repeating to himself, 'I think I can. I think I can. I think I can,' and when he finally crested the top of the big hill, he went down the other side saying, 'I knew I could. I knew I could. I knew I could!'"

Oddly enough, Daddy often tried to encourage me to think positive thoughts, a practice I have always tried to employ, and I appreciated his showing such concern for me during that difficult time.

Daddy's *other* personality was the polar opposite from the one we commonly saw, and it was one of the reasons I was conflicted in my feelings toward him.

After I had been placed in a regular hospital bed, I soon started using the open railing on the side of my bed to pull my arms through. I would garner all of my strength to hoist my weight against the bars, steadily increasing my arm strength each time.

As part of my therapy, I was given a hand strap to which the therapist attached a paintbrush so that I could paint whatever I wanted. As a girl, I had always loved to draw horses with a pencil, but I found that using paint was more fluid and easier to control than using a pencil. I now had a new hobby that brought me much satisfaction. I even painted a still life picture of a bowl of fruit of which I was very proud. I still have this painting and it is hanging on the wall in my youngest son's home with whom I am staying now.

With my new hobby, I began to think of all the other possibilities that awaited me once I returned home.

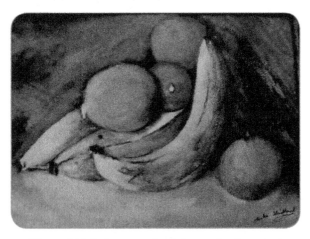

The still life I painted while in the hospital

Those who didn't believe my dream didn't live inside my head where I knew I had the power and control that, sooner or later, would help me keep the promise I had made to myself: I *would* walk out of the hospital on my own two legs. I also saw signs that I was even convincing some of my caretakers that my dream to walk was no illusion.

I began noticing that each of my hospital roommates was dying not long after being brought in. It became apparent to me that placing terminally ill patients in my room was done by design and purpose. Apparently the staff had noticed that I loved talking to people. I felt it was my God-given responsibility to help others when given the opportunity, even with my limited abilities. I did the best I knew how to do and hope that I made them feel better, even for such a short time.

There was one young man who had been brought into the hospital after a devastating motorcycle accident and had been placed in a room a few doors down from mine. He too had been diagnosed as a quadriplegic.

The parents of the young man—their only child—were deeply concerned because he was becoming withdrawn and seriously depressed. I knew exactly how he felt when he received his *death sentence*. There were times when I had felt the same way, but thankfully, I had pushed myself beyond that destructive way of thinking.

As part of my daily routine, I had begun ambulating up and down the hospital hallway in my wheelchair, talking to everyone I saw along the way. When any of my doctors saw me, they would smile and say, "Here comes our miracle patient."

I knew they weren't just giving me encouragement; I too had begun to believe that I had been given a miracle healing. I still had a long way to go before realizing my dream to walk again, but I tried to remain cheerful, looking only at the day in front of me.

I'm sure that it must have seemed strange when the boy's parents saw someone in my condition speaking to everyone with a smile on her face, always exuding such good cheer.

One day, the couple came into my room and asked if I could talk to their son because they seemed unable to say anything that made a difference in his will to live. Of course, I agreed! I was happy to have such a *mission*, one that allowed me the opportunity to help someone else and whose condition and frame of mind I completely understood.

I began to wheel myself down the hall to his room daily and always brought him a candy bar. I don't know if he welcomed my visits or was just being polite, but I continued to visit him and offer my encouragement.

The boy's parents often mentioned my cheerful attitude and had been hoping that some of it would rub off on their son, who still showed no interest in anything, including going to therapy. He had shut down emotionally and wanted no part of going through some "bogus" exercises that he believed would make little or no difference to his recovery.

Although I tried to share with him some of my optimism, I doubt it did much good.

With the help of many therapy sessions and my refusal to give up, I had begun to take a few steps with the aid of a walker. One day, I wheeled myself into the young man's hospital room, as I had always done, with candy in my hands, and said, "I'm going to deliver this candy to you, but not in the way I usually do." I raised up out of my wheelchair onto my feet, and with the aid of a walker and the strength of my upper arms, I walked to his bedside to deliver his treat.

The expression on the young man's face showed utter surprise, but I also believe that he never expected or dreamed of being able to walk again himself. I was slowly overcoming the most extreme odds, but we both knew that his chances of doing the same thing were probably far less than winning the lottery. I continued to be his friend and tried to give him the kind of encouragement I had always given myself. I was his greatest cheerleader and began to see his spirits improve as he began taking therapy on the tilt table.

I cannot fault anyone who feels that their life is over when they are lying in a hospital bed, day after day, looking back to a life that once was while fearing an unknown future. I just know that miracles really can and do happen. The last I heard about the young man's progress was that his attitude had improved, but after I left the hospital, I never learned what happened to him. I pray that he found spiritual understanding, a new purpose for his life, and a peaceful resolve. I do not say these things dismissively; I know how difficult the road ahead is for anyone like us.

## Coming Home…Almost

After several months, I was permitted to return home to be with my family on occasional weekends. What a blessing it was to be in my own home again, watching my children at play, not hampered by restrictive visiting hours. Don and I could talk at leisure, and I felt that life as I had known it before the accident could seamlessly resume once I was completely discharged from the hospital. Of course, I was aware of my limitations, but knowing how hard Don had pushed to keep the family together, I expected more of myself than perhaps I should have in those earlier days.

I wanted to act normal for my family and hoped for them to see me as their mother and wife without pity in their eyes. I wanted to do some of the household chores that would relieve Don of so many extra duties. God had greatly blessed me despite all that had happened, but I wanted even more now that I saw the results of my determination.

I would get my life back!

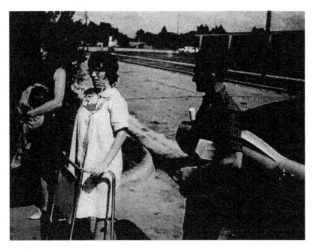

First trip home from the hospital wearing a neck brace—
but walking!
*Left,* sister-in-law Ruby; *right,* my husband, Don

## The Worst Trip Ever

It had been nearly a year since the accident. The time had finally come for me to leave the Wesley Medical Center Hospital and Wichita, Kansas, for good. I had had the most wonderful team of doctors, nurses, and therapists whom I believe the Lord had put there to help me through my long recovery. I owe each one of them a huge debt of gratitude. I had learned, although reluctantly, to lean completely on the help of others, and I had grown extremely humble through that experience. The Lord had never left my side, and I praise him for his constant love and tender care.

Don had asked to be reassigned to Langley Air Force Base in Hampton, Virginia, because it was near the home of my parents. In the event that Don was deployed to Vietnam, I would have the help and support of my parents while he was gone.

Because I was still a patient in transfer, I was not permitted to ride back to Virginia in the car with my husband and my children. I was placed on a stretcher and flown in a military hospital plane along with many soldiers who had been severely wounded in Vietnam that were headed to various hospitals, some to Langley AFB Hospital, with me. The stretchers were set up in three tiers, one on top of the other, and I could hear the agonizing moans and soft weeping of some of the worst wounded among them. There were only a few hospital attendants aboard, and they were probably doing their best to tend to the needs of those who needed help, but it wasn't enough. I know that the soldier above me had lost both of his legs because he and I talked throughout the plane trip.

I was heartsick as I heard the suffering and agonizing cries of these young wounded GIs, most of them in their early twenties, who had gone through and would continue to deal with the painful aftermath of war injuries long afterward—emotionally and physically. This was my worst experience since the accident. I had soiled myself, and there was no one to help any of us until we landed. I'm sure there were many others who felt as alone and humiliated as I did. When we finally landed, awaiting our second leg of the flight to Langley, we were taken to a large holding room (like cattle) where again there were not enough aides to administer to our needs. We remained in our own soiled clothing, feeling as though we were being punished for something we didn't understand. I remember crying to the Lord asking him to help all of us.

I remained at Langley hospital for a few months before I was allowed to go home on weekends as I had done in Wichita. The reason I had not yet been released to return home on a permanent basis was that I still had to rely on the use of catheters. The hospital tried various treatments designed to stimulate my bladder in preparation for my return home without further dependence on catheters. I was also shown exercises using my stomach muscles that eventually helped me to void a little on my own. Finally, the catheter was removed, and with the exception of regular outpatient therapy sessions, I was released from the hospital to finish my recovery at home.

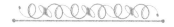

# Home at Last

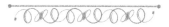

It felt like another lifetime ago that I had been a wife and mother to my family. I was scared. For an entire year, I had been under the constant care of others. What was my future going to be like? I felt like a stranger returning to a place where I had long ago belonged, but my role and purpose had now been eliminated or, at the very least, changed. I had looked so forward to this day, yet I wondered if I had prepared myself as well as I should have for the many changes that this new life would demand.

Don and I had previously rented the homes in which we lived, but we decided it was time to buy a house in Hampton, Virginia. We were fortunate to find a small house near Langley Air Force Base with a school for the children located right across the street from us. Everything we needed was in perfect proximity.

The house was very small, so Don converted the garage into our bedroom and placed inside the laundry facilities, my portable toilet, and other things that we needed for my care. Don was still taking care of all of my personal needs including my daily hygiene. He literally did everything for me as though I were a baby.

The fact that Don had to do such things made me worry about our husband-and-wife relationship. Much of my care was unpleasant and caused me a great deal of embarrassment.

I remember a time that we had driven to Langley AFB, and when walking back to the car, I felt my bowels involuntarily move (something that happened more times than I care to remember). There happened to be no place to take care of my needs, and I had to sit in my own mess until we returned home. This was only one of the many, many occasions that Don had to clean me up since I had no use of my hands. He never complained and never made me feel bad about these things. I will always be grateful to Don for his loving-kindnesses beyond what most people will ever be asked to do for a spouse.

Any woman reading this will probably cringe; however, I'm sure whether you are a man or woman, you can imagine how you would feel. There are things that we never want others to have to do for us. Notwithstanding the gratitude that follows, I believe the loss of this kind of privacy is the most difficult, especially if one maintains mental awareness.

We eventually got settled into our new home and began living as a family again. I could now take a few steps using a four-legged walker, which I used for many years. I would alternate between using the walker, the cane, and the wheelchair until I was finally able to use only crutches. I grew steadily stronger because of the workouts Don designed to help me rebuild my muscle strength.

Don pushed me pretty hard and would not allow me to use an excuse like, "I'm too tired." He insisted that I continue with my exercises so that I would not slip back from any progress I had already achieved. I never resented him for this because I knew he was helping me regain as much of my former life as I could manage.

Don was a military man with a strong personality, but I must give him tribute for all that he had purposed himself to do for me and the children. He was a great father and husband during the years we were together. We had many things to work out between us as husband and wife. I was home, but still unable to perform the tasks I had once done so effortlessly. Don and the children now did everything for me—they were wonderful—and we pulled together as best we could do.

I don't remember any instances where we were provided with home nursing, possibly because we were a military family, and I doubt that home care was provided through the military hospital. What this meant was that our family grew stronger because there was no one but ourselves to rely on. There was no one to counsel with us about our changed roles in the home, or how to manage our husband-and-wife relationship that would never be the same for either of us again.

As you might imagine, some of our biggest issues had to do with our intimate relationship. There were many sensitive issues we had to discuss and deal with that I must touch on here because they may be relevant to some of my readers.

Don was a normal man with a wife who could no longer feel his caresses. This bothered him more than he wanted me to know, as I'm certain it would for any man who is sensitive to his wife's feelings.

I tried to convince Don that physical arousal was generated in the brain anyway, and I wanted him to stop worrying and feeling guilty. He was my husband, and I honestly wanted him to continue sharing his affections for and with me. Although I had lost all feeling in my lower body, I was still able to enjoy a continued deep emotional response to his tenderness.

Another related problem was that I unfortunately still relied on the use of catheters after I returned home from the hospital. Since I had no use of my hands, Don had to learn how to change them—another loss of dignity for me and another added burden for Don.

I was becoming a bit more able to manage some of the household chores by using my cane to get around, and I was determined to assume as many duties around the house as I could reasonably manage.

There was a beauty shop a couple of doors down from our house, and I would walk there to have them wash my hair so that Don wouldn't have to do that too. I want to emphasize that Don didn't complain about the extra work, but, at times, I could feel his frustration. All I wanted to do was take some of the load off him.

Being back at home was a blessing, but I became aware that my life was more altered than my optimistic thoughts had previously permitted me to consider. Everything required an adjustment of one kind or another, and Don rallied again by creating some of the most innovative tools and devices to help me do things that I would not have been able to do without them.

Some of the inventions Don made to help me perform my tasks are now being used in hospitals for patients with my type of injuries. Had Don patented those homemade inventions before they had been discovered by others, he would have become a very wealthy man.

One of the inventions Don made for me might not solicit much admiration from my readers, but, in a very practical manner, it was important. Without the use of my hands, it was sometimes difficult to discipline the children, who could really take advantage of my situation. So Don made a leather strap that held a tree switch to swat the occasional mischievous bottom if warranted. To some, this will seem amusing; to others, it may seem audacious; but anyone who has raised five children will understand that, by sheer numbers, I was at a distinct disadvantage, especially in my condition.

I gradually became familiar with our new neighborhood in Hampton and got to know my next-door neighbor, a kind and loving Italian woman who often came over to our house before dinnertime to help me get my evening meal started. She would put the spaghetti on or do other things that I found difficult. I will never forget her kindness so many years ago when it meant so much.

Our family worked hard together, everyone doing regular chores to keep the household running as smoothly as possible, but we also played together. We enjoyed camping, picnicking, and going to the beach. It was wonderful to get outside and smell the fragrances of spring and summer. We found many activities that we could enjoy without spending a lot of money.

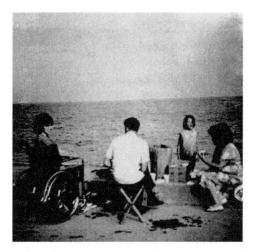

A trip to the beach while visiting Canada with the family

I was able to enjoy these outings because I felt more alive when I was out in nature; however, these events were not without their dangers. I remember a certain picnic where all of my kids wanted to go down to fish at the lake after lunch. The lake was not far from the picnic table where we had set up, but no one felt comfortable leaving me alone because at the time, I couldn't walk yet. I told them that I would be fine and asked them just to set me on the ground by the tree and to go have some fun. So Don and the kids helped me out of my wheelchair and set me in a nice spot on the ground under a big shady tree. While Don and the kids were fishing, all of a sudden an army of ants started crawling all over me. At first I tried to swat them away with my hands, but there were too many of them, and I started yelling for help. Thank goodness they heard me and came running to my rescue!

I recall another time when I had to go to the restroom and my family helped me get to the door but left me alone to go inside because by this time, I was able to use a walker. I'm sure they thought I would be able to manage, but when I was finished and ready to leave, I couldn't open the restroom door and was trapped inside. I panicked and began to scream for help. Of course, they all came running.

These are the types of anecdotes that illustrate my dependence upon others. Even though I had some increased mobility, I never knew when I might find myself in a situation that I couldn't manage by myself.

Since our first house was so small, Don and I decided to look for a bigger one that would accommodate our growing children. We found a lovely home in a nice neighborhood, and we were all excited to move into a house where we had more room. I was also gaining more mobility, and my overall health was steadily improving. It was during the time that we lived in our new home that Don received orders to go to Vietnam. I know he was very worried about leaving me, but I knew I would be fine since we now lived close to other family members, and my children could not have been more helpful; they were always there for me and so willing to help, no matter what it was that I needed.

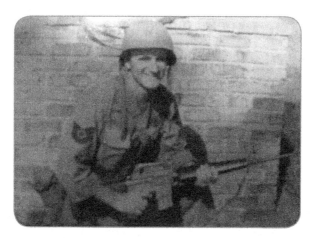

Don Widlacki during his tour in Vietnam

I received a phone call from my father after Don left for Vietnam, and he said that he and my mother were going to come for a visit. It was on this very rare occasion that I gained enough nerve to tell him that, though I loved him and wanted them to visit, I had to insist that he come to visit dressed as a man, not as a woman (which he had begun to do more frequently). I cried during the entire phone conversation because I knew he was growing very angry with me. He hung up the phone and did not speak to me for at least a year, and neither of my parents came to visit during that time.

While Don was gone, I also started driving a car again because of my father's encouragement before the fated phone call. But when Don found out, he expressed deep concern for my safety and the safety of our children due to my obvious physical limitations.

The doctors could not believe my progress. Here I was, not only walking but driving too. I had even begun babysitting for neighbors with the help of my children.

## Home from Vietnam, 1971

The children and I were so excited when Don finally came home after a year in Vietnam, but things didn't feel the same between us. When Don came inside the house, the children were standing stair-step fashion and sang a song I had taught them from the movie *The Sound of Music*. He seemed delighted with their performance and greeted each of them warmly, but he hardly paid any attention to me, and our communications immediately felt strained.

I know that Don's year away from home must have provided him a great deal of time to consider how his life had changed since my accident; perhaps he had enjoyed his freedom away from the demands of our home so much so that he no longer wanted to deal with all of it—especially with me and my constant needs. Previously, Don had been fairly good at controlling his feelings, yet I saw and felt his frustrations early on and watched helplessly as they began to manifest in stronger ways.

A couple of years after my accident, Don had driven me to one of my doctor's appointments, and for some reason, he and the doctor got into a heated argument that embarrassed me so much that I walked out of the doctor's office into the hallway. Don and the doctor followed right behind me, and I heard the doctor yelling at my husband saying, "My God, man, she should be six feet under the ground or still in the wheelchair, and you're complaining? You should be thankful because your wife is a walking miracle!"

Despite the fact that our relationship was changing, Don and I went on trying to make the best of our situation. Don remained in the Air Force, but we began dabbling in real estate for extra money.

I had always wanted a lot of land since I had grown up in rural Virginia, and I still preferred a bucolic life to that of living in the city. I discovered that Don felt exactly the opposite; he wanted to live in an urban community, in an established neighborhood.

I found a small house on five acres of land, and though Don didn't like the property, he agreed to buy it for my sake and that of our children. The children and I loved our new home in the country. We cleared a portion of the land so that we could eventually build a nice house on it, and we bought the children a pony. I raised dogs, and we also had some goats and several cats because the children loved all kinds of animals as much as I did. I am very grateful that my love for animals, since childhood, has carried over to my own children.

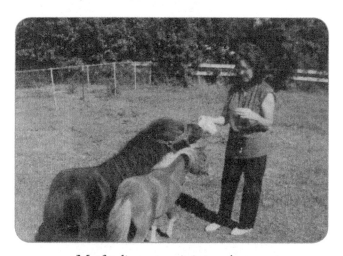

Me feeding my miniature horses

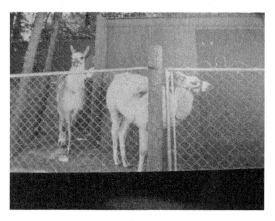

My llamas

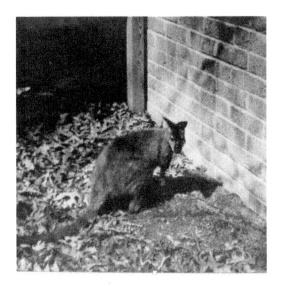

Pet joey

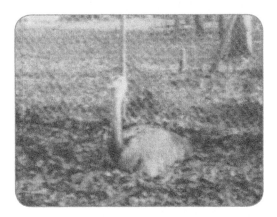

Pet emu

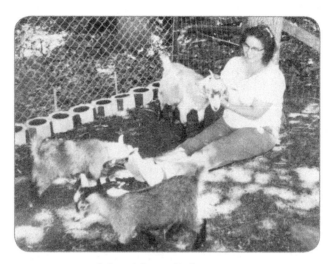

Me with my little goats

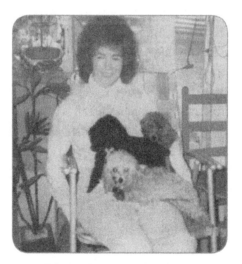

Me with a few of my dogs

*Julia Dean Childress Widlacki*

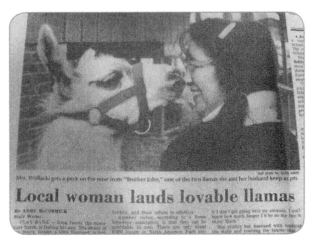

Newspaper clipping of me with my pet llama, Brother John

I can't remember a time when we didn't have a house and/or yard full of dogs, cats, snakes, monkeys, goats, kangaroos, miniature horses, and llama. We also had birds, lizards, guinea pigs, white fox, to name a few more. I wish I could say that Don shared the children's and my enthusiasm for our growing menagerie, but he was never bitten (pun intended) by that particular interest. He did, however, build many pens, cages, fences, and corrals for them on our five-acre farm, so I can't fault him for not trying. Having animals was a big part of our lives, and like everything else that we shared, it drew us closer because of the joy we received in caring for them together. I have some wonderful, lasting memories of our beloved family pets; each has gained a special place in my heart.

My youngest son, Guy, recalls some amusing stories about our pet squirrel monkey; one in particular still makes us laugh.

We had all piled into the car for a family outing when in our upstairs window, we saw the monkey perched up on a bed watching us from the window. He was fervently licking a Tootsie Pop lollipop as he saw us drive away, and we all got a good laugh out of it. When we came home much later in the day, the monkey was still sitting at the window licking the lollipop, but his tongue must have gotten tired because by then, he was licking the lollipop in slow motion and had almost gotten to the Tootsie Roll center.

The monkey also liked to crush the toilet paper rolls in the bathroom and did many other mischievous deeds. I don't know how many times we had to take one of the children to the doctor's office for a tetanus shot because he had bitten them. I thought it was prudent to ask the doctor to give all the kids a preventative tetanus shot, but he said he couldn't do that until they had actually been bitten. (I still think my own logic was the best line of defense.)

We worked diligently to train that little monkey to behave, and we also got him to wear diapers, but we eventually had to get rid of him because he wouldn't give up his habit of biting the children. I believe whoever got that little rascal after we had trained him got a much better monkey than the one we started with.

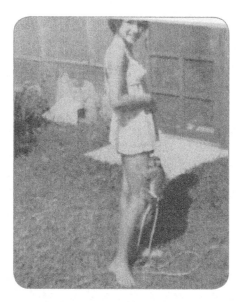

Susie, age 9, and our "rascal" monkey

We also acquired a pair of wild rhesus monkeys that were offered to us with the proviso that we had to "catch them first"—not an easy feat since those monkeys were smart little devils. Once we got them, and because they were wild, we had to keep them away from people.

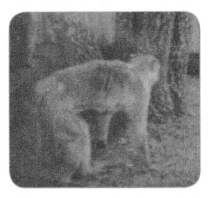

Rhesus monkeys in cage Don built

Don again built another extravagant cage the size of an average room. One of our young visiting relatives got too near the cage, and one of the monkeys pulled out a chunk of his hair. We eventually had to get rid of those pets too because the male was vicious to the female and continued to bite her. We later found out that they were brother and sister and would not mate for that reason. But we gave them to a zoo, and hopefully they had the freedom to enjoy life among their peers.

Over the years, we had many dogs, and one was quite vicious. We heard that he had been a show dog that had been mistreated. I believe he was a mix between husky and Alaskan malamute, and for some reason, we were never able to train him.

I have to admit that along with our naughty little monkey, that dog caused us a lot of vet bills, and once he even castrated one of our goats. This dog could look so friendly, but it was difficult to read his intentions. Guy went down on his knees to pet him one day, and when he got too close, the dog snapped and put Guy's whole face in his mouth. I always liked to think that I could train any problem animal, but I was wrong about this one. The man who eventually bought the dog seemed pleased that he would snap and bite. We have no idea what the man's plans for the dog were, but this one would have made a perfect junkyard dog.

After Don had been sent to Vietnam, the children and I sort of went overboard with animals. I probably would have had to classify our collection at that time as a small zoo; we even had a talking mynah bird.

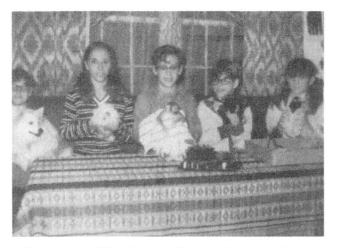

*Left to right:* Tim, Donna, Donny, Guy, and Susie

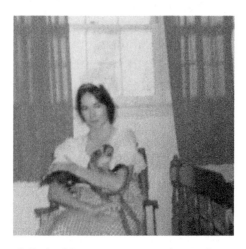

Me holding our squirrel monkey

The children had to help me even more than usual with Don away; they had to do everything needed for running a household that I was unable to do. I tried to take turns calling on each of the children so that I didn't rely too much on any one of them. Well, the mynah bird got so used to hearing me call for Donna (my oldest daughter) that he would also call her name, and she would come running upstairs, or downstairs, depending on where I was, thinking it was me who had called her. It was then that I realized that I must have been calling on Donna far too much for the mynah bird to have learned her name over that of the other children!

Our whole family worked hard to improve the five-acre property. The children worked outside every day when they got home from school, and they loved the work. They decided that they wanted to dam up the underground streams to make a small lake that took a year and a half to accomplish. They also cut logs from the woods, cut off the branches, stripped the bark, and made a fenced corral for the horses.

Don was never happy in the country, so, in fairness to him, we moved again two years later to a city neighborhood. While we lived in this new home, Don was getting ready to retire from the Air Force, and he became more involved in real estate as a way to supplement his retirement income.

When Don and I were out looking for some property in which to invest, I stepped in a hole and broke my ankle. I never felt the injury occur because I was still without feeling in my legs and feet, but when my leg began to swell, I was taken to the hospital where they put on a cast that went all the way from my ankle to my knee. This made my mobility even more difficult, so I decided to go back to school to get my high school diploma, which I had never done because I had married before my high school graduation.

The rules of my high school forbade me to continue attending school since I had become pregnant in the last part of my senior year. I had been able to attend my prom and other activities but was not able to get my diploma—something that had always bothered me. All that was required for me to graduate was English 12, literature, and grammar, and it had been my intention to pay for my own tutoring and finish my graduation requirements during the summer school session of the year I was supposed to graduate. However, at the time I had intended to begin my tutoring, Don's four-year stint in the Navy had been completed, and he had joined the Air Force. The money I had saved from selling my horse would have paid for my classes, but we used the money for the cross-country move to Wichita Falls, Texas, instead. After that, we were relocated three more times before being stationed in Japan. When we arrived back in the States, we were stationed in Wichita, Kansas, where our lives began to spiral out of control.

So with my latest injury and a cumbersome cast on my leg, I finally attended night school and received my high school diploma. I was thrilled with my newest accomplishment, and it didn't matter how long it had taken me to reach this milestone,

I had, with the help of God, achieved one more important goal that I had set out to do.

Our family moved again after finding a lovely home on the water. Since Don loved to fish, it seemed to be a perfect location for us.

Don built the children a recreation room so that they could have a place to entertain their many friends, and I loved seeing everyone happy.

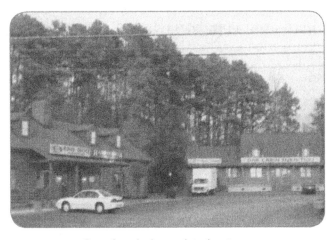

Our family log cabin business

It was during this time that our real estate business started to boom. We had started our own company that manufactured and sold log cabin homes. This was a prosperous time for us; we all worked together in the family business and enjoyed a great deal of success.

Time flew by with work and our many activities, and soon our children were, one by one, graduating from high school and getting ready to leave for college and other life adventures. One followed in Don's footsteps and went into the US Navy, three of them went on to college, and one decided to get married. This seemed like a good time for me to go back to school and get my real estate license so that I could be of more help to Don with our growing real estate business. It was difficult; I was terrible in math, but Don taught me how to work the math problems that I would encounter when I took the licensing exam.

I was still on crutches at the time, but I didn't let that stop me from achieving my goal. When it came time to take the test, I could tell that Don was concerned that I might not be able to do the math calculations. After the exam, I nervously awaited the test results. I listened daily for the postman to deliver the news as to whether I had or hadn't passed. When the envelope with my results finally arrived, the anticipation was almost too much for my heart. I think I was trembling when I read that *I had passed!*

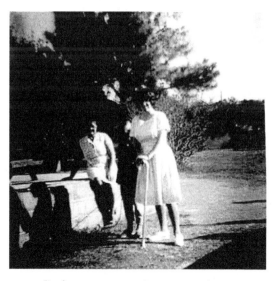

Before my second auto accident,
I walked with only the use of a cane.

# A Storm Strikes Again

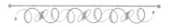

It had been ten years since the accident that had caused my broken neck. Although lightning isn't supposed to strike twice in the same place, I had become accustomed to living my life against the odds. As unbelievable as it may seem, I was involved in a second automobile accident. This time, however, I was a passenger, and since there were no seat belt restraints in the car, I had been thrown forward from the backseat to the front of the car and smashed my left knee. I required three surgeries prior to my total left knee replacement. Talk about insult to injury!

I became even more dependent upon Don and my children for my day-to-day care. I was hospitalized again and felt as though I had slid backward from all of my progress and hard work. During my recovery, I went back to using my wheelchair, walker, and crutches whereas I had previously only been using a cane to get around.

I felt terrible! My family had endured many burdens with my day-to-day, ongoing care; now everything had gotten worse. While I was in another long-term recovery, it became impossible for me to exercise, my bladder had stopped functioning properly, and I had difficulty voiding. I was subsequently put into a bladder training program that took months to achieve, during which time Don and my oldest daughter, Donna, (again) had to help me with the use of catheters. I witnessed the strain that all of this extra work was putting on my family, especially on Don, but I was helpless to do anything to change the situation.

The emotional distance between Don and me steadily grew. I knew that Don had done everything possible for my care and special needs, but I also knew he was worn out from the problems that seemed to multiply faster than we could solve them. The only thing we could do was put up a happy front and deal with life as it came.

In an attempt to help our marriage during these times of increased demands on me, Don, and the children, we had decided to have a little celebration for our twenty-fifth wedding anniversary. We chose to have it in one of the log cabins on the log cabin complex that Don and the children helped to build. This "new beginning," however, lasted only a short while.

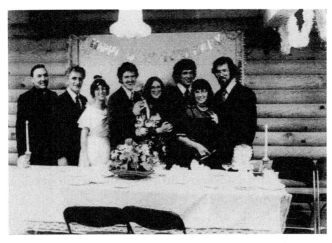

25th Wedding Anniversary with family and Father Quinn; from left to right: Father Quinn, Don, Donna, Timmy, Susie, Guy, me/mom, and Donnie.

As the children began to grow up and leave, Don and I didn't need the large house we had been living in when they were all at home, so we decided to find a smaller one. This time, I found a house I thought would make Don happy. As I have mentioned before, he preferred living in a neighborhood surrounded by other people, and I enjoyed the exact opposite. The house I found seemed, to me, a fair compromise that would make us both happy. There was enough land for me to enjoy being outdoors with room for my animals, and it was situated in a structured neighborhood, backed by a lake.

I thought Don was happy with the house since he had signed the mortgage papers, and after we had moved in, he worked very hard on improvements and even built a very nice boathouse.

It wasn't long though before Don became restless and seemed to find fault with, among other things, the noise level around our property. When Don was unhappy, I always felt responsible because of the burden I had become to him. I tried to do many things to help him and had purchased an electric lawnmower so that I could help him keep up with the yard maintenance.

One day while I was helping Don in the yard, he seemed to be in a bad mood and showed very little patience with me. When we had finished our work and had come back inside the house, both of us exhausted, I tried to figure out what to fix for our dinner. For no apparent reason, Don became very upset with me and walked out of the house. After a while, he returned and said that he was leaving me.

I was heartbroken. I had tried so hard to help Don and did everything I knew how to do in order to keep our marriage together, but Don was fed up.

## Brother Clyde to the Rescue Again

It was around this time that my brother Clyde and his lovely wife, Connie, invited Don and me to visit them at their home in Southern California. Clyde had thoughtfully invited another couple who were dealing with the same kinds of problems that Don and I were, except that the husband was a diagnosed quadriplegic, and his wife was his caretaker—the exact reverse of our circumstances.

Although it was a wonderful trip and very cathartic to have another couple with whom to share some of the same issues and difficulties that Don and I had, very little change occurred between Don and me upon returning home.

I truly love my brother for all of his kindnesses and the heartfelt compassion that he has exhibited toward me and so many others. He lives a committed Christian life dedicated to helping as many people who come into his life as he possibly can.

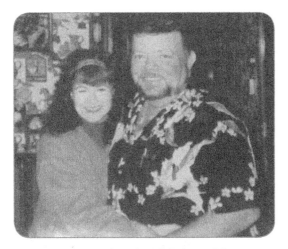

My big brother Clyde and I

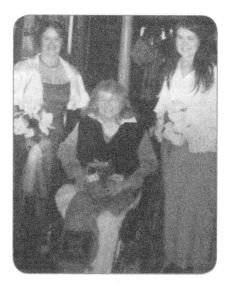

*Left,* my sister Sherry; *middle,* me; *right,* my sister Connie
(Recent picture was taken at my brother
Clyde's home for Sherry's wedding)

I had seen Don's attitude toward me changing for quite some time. The distance between us was palpable as his personal unhappiness became more evident in the way he spoke to me and in his lack of patience over things he had once done for me without complaint or resentment. Don wanted to leave; I had no more cards in my hands left to play. I was now forced to deal with life alone, with a myriad of complications associated with my disability. I often fell, and without help, it was almost impossible for me to get up by myself.

One day as I was walking out of the shower, my toe caught on something, and I tripped and fell hard onto the floor. I tried to steady myself with my right arm, but I had no strength. I couldn't lift my legs since I had no feeling in my limbs, especially my left leg with the knee replacement from the last car accident. I pushed hard onto my right arm, but it kept going backward, and I could hear it snap and break then dislocate from the socket. I gathered every bit of my waning strength and slowly scooted my body across the floor to our office to call for help. I was in such a bad state of mind that I could hardly think of whom to call. There had always been people around me, and this was the first time I had found myself completely alone.

I called my oldest daughter, Donna, who came over immediately to help me get up off the floor. I had forgotten that all of the outside doors were locked, but somehow she got to me quickly and drove me to the hospital. The first thing they did was put my dislocated arm back in place, and not for the first time, I was glad that my limbs had no feeling. Next, they put my arm in a sling but could not cast it due to the way in which I had broken it.

I really had a dilemma now. I had no feeling in my left hand and no use of my right arm. With my latest injury, I would have even more difficulty taking care of myself even performing the most minimal activities such as getting dressed.

Ever since the first automobile accident had rendered me a quadriplegic, I have had so many setbacks that I've lost count. As soon as I had managed to solve one issue, another one would surface, often worse than the previous one. I seemed to have been on a fast track to my own demise, and I had no idea where it would end. But, one thing is certain, whatever trials were placed in front of me, I foraged ahead with the certain knowledge that the Lord and I would somehow get me through all of it.

I eventually had to sell our house, and Donna helped me find a nice place to rent. I had signed a one-year lease on the rental house eventually expecting to purchase it. Had I stayed, the house would have been a very good buy, but I wasn't thinking straight and decided to ask the owner if I could get out of my lease. The landlord said that if I could find someone to take over my lease, he would allow me to get out of it, which I did.

Sadly, I had to sell all of my animals except for my little miniature horse and some dogs. I bought a little house on an acre of land, which turned out to be one of the worst investments I had ever made. I know that my poor decisions had to do with heartache over the divorce that I didn't want and having to sell the home that I had enjoyed so much with my family.

I learned that it is fruitless to become attached to the things of this world; we will not take anything with us except for our deeds, our knowledge, the love we have for each other, and whatever degree of faith in the Lord we have attained. Everything else pales in comparison.

# More Than Enough!

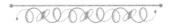

When a truly tragic event happens in our lives, a litany of nagging questions run through our minds that help us sort through the facts (as we understand them) in order to make spiritual sense of it. I needed to understand God's purpose for me and why I had to be in a severely handicapped body in order to perform the mission that he had set before me.

A thought occurred to me—a foolish one, as I look back—that nothing worse could happen to me because of all the difficult things I had already endured. I felt insulated because surely God knew that I had experienced enough tragedy for one lifetime, so I thought God, in his mercy, certainly had to know that enough was enough—didn't he?

I've been told that God does not give us more than we can bear, and if that truly is the case, he must have already prepared my spirit for the next great upheaval. The idea that God holds back from teaching a crucial life lesson seems (to me) like whistling in the dark in order to make ourselves feel invincible while we are shaking in our shoes.

I now believe that God is most willing to send a lightning bolt to pierce a rebellious heart rather than allow that soul to be eternally lost, as it is written in Hebrews 12:6 (St. Jerome's

Catholic Study Bible), "For whom the Lord loveth he chasteneth, and scourgeth every son whom he receiveth."

My thoughts may be somewhat subjective on these matters, and there are those who will disagree with my observations, but all of us are entitled to our own personal revelations.

I have no anger or resentment toward God for any- and everything that has happened to me, only gratitude for the light that has followed the darkness.

I have sustained other deep hurts and losses over the years, not the least of which was Don asking for a divorce so that he could marry a woman without the handicaps that plagued our lives and kept me from being the kind of wife that Don needed. I was devastated, but how could I blame him? Don had given all he felt he could give, and he needed more for his own happiness.

About a year before Don left me (the first time), God had given me a dream vision where the Lord Jesus stood at the top of a beautiful golden stairway with angels flanking each side. As I looked up at the Lord, his arms were outstretched toward me. He wore a white robe with a blue sash and was surrounded by a brilliant light that shone all around him. I was at the bottom of the stairs, looking up, and heard the Lord say to me, "Do not be afraid. I give you my peace. I will always be with you. I love you, my daughter. Take one step at a time, step over one obstacle at a time. You will be all right." Then I awoke and was in awe trying to figure out what had just happened, because the dream was so real, which is how I knew I had received a vision. My life's trials were not over. I did not understand it at the time, but in looking back, I have come to understand what he meant.

Don started going out with a woman with whom he could do all kinds of activities that he could no longer do with me. I tried to convince him that, with a few modifications, he and I could do more of those same things together. I even telephoned the woman who Don had been seeing and asked her to "Please, leave my husband alone." But she refused. She informed me that she and Don would be getting married once he had met and accepted her children and they him.

These events began a yearlong soap opera. Don kept pushing me to sign the divorce papers, and I kept refusing. Finally, in February 1987, Don had succeeded in weakening my resolve to keep our marriage intact, but I signed the papers against my wishes.

When I left the lawyer's office, Don was outside waiting for me, and I asked, "What are you doing here, making sure I signed the papers?"

He said, "No, I just want us to have a cup of coffee together and talk."

So we talked about his plans to meet his girlfriend's children the following day, and we still communicated with each other quite often after that.

For my part, I was just trying my best to get my husband back, but for Don's, I believe he just wanted to make sure that I was doing okay while he was still seeing the *other woman*.

## Until Death Do We Part…Again

By the end of the year, my efforts must have paid off because Don came to me and said that he felt the Lord wanted us to be remarried.

As incredible as it seemed, and as elated as I was, I asked Don, "Are you sure?" and he said yes, but a nagging little voice inside my head kept asking the most important question: Was his decision to remarry me motivated by guilt, compassion, or genuine love? I was so excited about remarrying my beloved husband that I did not let my concerns override my joy. Don and I remarried at the end of that year, on December 22, the same date we had gotten married thirty-three years before.

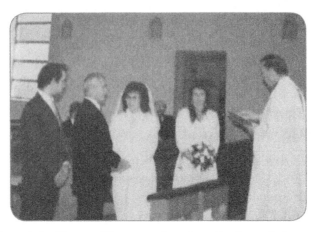

*Left to right:* Donny, Don, me, daughter Susie, and the pastor
Our remarriage ceremony

On the night that we got remarried, I had dressed up very nicely expecting that we would go out to celebrate, but my husband would not have anything to do with my wishes. He said there was no way he was going out and that if I wanted to go somewhere, I could go by myself. His words and attitude hurt me very much and caused me to question why he had married me again after he was free.

I did, as I had always done and tried to make the best of the situation, I got dressed for bed in a pretty negligee and went to show Don how I looked. I walked over to where he sat on the bed and gave him a hug. When he hugged me back, he said, "You feel mushy," and he wouldn't have anything to do with me that night.

The next morning when we got up, I fixed Don a nice breakfast hoping that the day would go better. The phone rang as we were getting ready to sit down at the table, and I answered the call.

A woman's voice asked for Don; it was the woman he had been dating prior to our divorce! I asked her for the second time to leave my husband alone and allow us to work on our marriage.

It was about a month into our remarriage that I finally faced the fact that Don's heart was not really into it, but I knew that he had been trying, and I really appreciated him for making an effort. It became apparent that Don was torn between trying to make our marriage work and his girlfriend's efforts to pull him away because they had continued to see each other after we were remarried.

Don asked for a second divorce, but I told him that I was not going to sign any divorce papers again. I also told him that if he wanted a divorce, he would have to do it without my help. Don was very distraught and angry at this and had actually admitted himself into the hospital. After that, we began seeing marriage therapists.

The first therapist whom we met asked Don a question, to which Don replied, "I like to hold a firm hand." At that time, I could not use my right hand very well, and I could not use my left hand at all (even to this day). The doctor told Don that his comment was an awful thing to say. I know that Don felt his own happiness slipping further and further away, and he began to dwell only upon the negatives in our marriage.

The doctor turned to me and asked me to describe how Don's words had made me feel. I confessed that hearing Don say such things hurt me, but I understood where he was coming from. The doctor gave me a rather stern look and asked me why I would still want to stay with a man who said such careless and thoughtless things. I gave the only answer I could give—the truth. I said that I loved Don and didn't believe in divorce and that I was hoping, with God's help, we might still be able to work through our difficulties and save our marriage.

Don and I went to a few more therapists after that, but each time my husband would walk out before the sessions were over, and I would be left in the therapists' offices crying. Each therapist asked me the same question: "Why do you want to remain in this marriage?"

I guess I was being stubborn and slow to realize that a marriage requires two people who both want to make it work. For some reason, I was unable to grasp the idea that Don simply wanted to leave. I grew to understand that Don had agreed to attend therapy in order to make it *appear* that he had done everything he could do to help save our marriage before he actually walked out. Don certainly must have known how it would have looked to our family and friends. He didn't want to be viewed as a coward, and he wasn't. I know he tried very hard—sometimes more than others—and I do not hold anything against him because his life was shattered just as much as mine was. Although Don's attitude hurt me, I know that he was hurting too. My heart went out to him because neither one of us knew how to help the other. I realized then that you cannot change someone else's will, only your own.

After Mother's Day that year, Don's girlfriend got her own divorce, and he wanted to marry her. Since I would not sign the divorce papers, he came out to where I was living in Gloucester and threatened my life.

I know that Don's emotions got the best of him after I refused (again) to sign the divorce papers. I truly was not trying to get back at my husband. I just knew that I had given him a divorce once before, and I was not going to sign divorce papers a second time. Since I don't believe in divorce, I honestly felt that we could have at least tried to work things out between us, and I just did not realize how upset he was over the entire situation. If only Don had been willing to wait a year, he could have had the divorce without my signature, but he wasn't willing to wait. I just wanted to be left out of it because I still truly loved him even after all that he had put me through.

Don's girlfriend was free at the time, and he wanted to marry her without waiting, so he kept pressing me to sign the papers. Because I would not, he left the house in anger. Later that same day, I heard a knock at my door, and when I opened it, there stood my husband with a suitcase in one hand and a six-pack of beer in the other. He was completely drunk, which frightened me because I knew what it was like to be around him when he was drinking. Considering his condition, I tried to prevent him from coming in the house, but he pushed me aside, walked right in, and yelled, "Well, your husband is home, and I will show you what *hell* is all about!"

I was no match for his strength. He pushed me up against the wall and, in an angry tone, said, "Fix me something to eat." I quickly grabbed a can of stew and started fixing it on the stove, but while I was busy doing this, he kicked my dog.

I said in a scared tone, "Don't do that!" I rushed to put my dog in her cage to protect her from his rage and went back to the stove, and he threw beer on the floor where I stood. As soon as he did that, I turned off the stove, got my purse, and tried my best to walk out of the house. Keeping in mind that I was very slow and was using a crutch, I somehow managed to get down the front porch steps with him in close pursuit. When he caught up with me, he jerked my purse off my shoulder and threw it down by the car. Then he tossed beer all over me, from the top of my head to my feet, before lunging at me with a knife. I said, "Stop it! What is wrong with you?" But he didn't stop and tried to come after me again.

All of a sudden, a tall, blond-haired young man just happened to appear and walked right in front of us. This gave me the courage to scream and shout, "Please call the police! My husband is trying to kill me!" This distracted my husband, and he went back inside the house, allowing me to get to the road where I tried flagging down a car. I turned to say thank you to the young man, but he had just disappeared. What puzzled me about the appearance of this young man was that we were out in the country and no one lived near our home. I tried to figure out where he had gone, but I was so upset from the incident that I continued flagging cars until one stopped. The kind person who stopped took me to the country store down the road where I knew the owner, and when he saw me, he said, "What in the world happened to you?" I related all that had happened and said I was not going back to the house. The owner said that I should call the police, but I didn't want to, so he called them.

When the police came, I told them everything. One of the policemen saw the cross that I wore around my neck and asked, "Are you Catholic?"

I answered, "Yes, but that has nothing to do with my decision. I just do not personally believe in divorce." I also explained that I did not want to sign the divorce papers again and described in detail the events that had led to my husband's abusive behavior. They asked me if I wanted to press charges, and when I told them that I preferred not to, they asked if I had anywhere else to stay that night. I told them that I could stay with my oldest daughter down the road. They told me to get in their car and that they would take me back to my house to get some things I needed. I was afraid, but they assured me nothing would happen to me with them there to protect me. When we got to the house, I proceeded to get the items I needed. My husband was being really silly asking all kinds of questions. The police said that I did not have to answer him. When I had finished packing, they took me to my daughter Donna's house and advised me not to let my husband on her property. After we arrived, Donna called her father (my husband) and told him that what he had done was a terrible thing to do to me. He told her that he had not intended to hurt me and was only trying to scare me. I believe she responded with, "It was a *bad* way to go about it." The next morning, I asked Donna to take me back to my house, and I was relieved to find that my husband had gone back to his own house. I know that he was very upset and hurt over the entire incident, and what he really wanted was his freedom to marry and not have to wait another year.

When I was back at home contemplating all that had happened, I came to believe that it was an angel who had come to save me the previous day. It must have been an angel who intervened because there was no one else around, and he appeared as quickly as he had disappeared. I thank God for this.

I can't blame Don because of the decline of our marriage. Sometimes I think it's harder on the mate who is not afflicted than on the one who is impaired. I know that Don stuck it out as long as he felt he could stay without completely ignoring his own happiness. I often saw Don struggle with his conscience. I know he was engaged in a heated war between what he needed for himself and his desire to do the right thing for me.

One occasion that best illustrates his ongoing conflict after my second accident is the time when he refused to go with me to our older son Donny's graduation from boot camp in Florida. Don had been drinking that day and did not want to participate. He knew that I wanted to go, but I became frightened of his actions and told him that I would stay home too. Don grew adamant and actually made me go. I was scared because I was using the walker at the time, and I had never flown by myself before. Don made me pack my suitcase, drove me to the airport, and made me get on the plane. Everybody was so nice, and I should have known that the Lord would be watching over me as he always had. My confidence was renewed as the flight went on without any problems. I attended my son's boot camp graduation the next morning. After the beautiful ceremony, Donny asked where his Dad was. I told him that I could not get him to come. The more I thought about Don refusing to attend his own son's graduation, the more upset I grew and told Donny that I was not going to go home. Donny was compassionate and understood my feelings, but he eventually convinced me to go back and said that he would go back with me. When we arrived at the airport back home, I found out that Don had been at the airport all day checking every flight that had come from Florida. We didn't know that he was waiting at the airport because I never told Don our flight number. But when Don saw me, he ran over and hugged me and told me that he was so sorry and that he loved me. So we went home and started again. This is just a few examples of the on-again-off-again conflicts that took place as we struggled to keep our marriage going for as long as we did. I know Don's life was in as much turmoil as mine was, and he often showed remorse for acting out his feelings in a way that hurt me.

Fate can often be cruel. I received my second divorce papers on Valentine's Day. I asked the policeman who delivered them. "Couldn't you have waited until tomorrow to serve these papers?" I spent the entire day crying and praying. The second divorce really devastated me—I believe even more so than did my accident.

Following that very unsettling incident with Don when (I believe) an angel saved me from his rage, we had not spoken of it until the end of the year when my father died. Don came to the funeral to pay his respects and informed me that our divorce had been finalized the previous day. I didn't say anything about it; I just told him that I was going to live with my mother because she had asked me to move in with her.

Watching Don walk out of my life for the last time was more painful than all of the things I had endured up to that point. I saw my entire history with the young man I had loved from the days of my youth fade like an old photograph as he left me standing there wondering what would become of me, of us.

As I turned around, who should I meet (again) at my father's funeral but an old friend, Doug Newcomb, whom I had known many years prior when we were both teenagers.

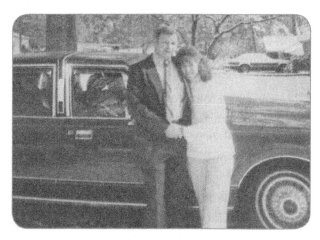

My friend Doug Newcomb and me

While living with my mother, Doug and I became reacquainted because he was also single. We grew to be the best of friends, and he helped me through a lot of bad times by allowing me to talk to him about my ex-husband. I really want to thank him for this because when a person is grieving, sometimes all that anyone can do to help is just listen.

It is really wonderful how the Lord puts someone in your pathway that fulfills what you need at the time. Doug is a really wonderful man, and we remain good friends to this day.

Initially, when my mother asked me to move in with her, I had to pray about the decision because I had made a spiritual commitment to join the sisterhood of nuns in Florida. As I prayed about it, I felt that the Lord was leading me to stay with my mother so that I could be of help to her as her health had been slowly declining.

### More Surgeries

During the time that I lived with my mother, the retina in my right eye had become detached and I went blind in that eye, but the doctors were able to save my sight. In 1990, the doctors diagnosed me with hepatitis C; in 1992, I had a C4 vertebra fused, and in 1993, I had cataract surgery in both eyes, and later, a left knee replacement from the second car accident (more on that later).

A while later, I had to have another knee surgery, but this time it was on my right knee. As I was recuperating and still feeling the postoperative effects, my daughter Donna mentioned that she felt a doctor should see me as she sensed something was wrong. When the doctor came to check on me, he found that my artery had accidentally been cut during the knee surgery, and I almost bled to death.

God had again intervened. The best vascular surgeon in the area just happened to be at the hospital (he was not on duty at the time) and immediately performed the corrective surgery that kept me from bleeding to death. One of the orthopedic doctors said that angels must have surely been watching over me.

On another occasion, I had burned both of my feet with second-degree burns after stepping into a pool of scalding water from my broken hot water heater. Although I had no feeling in my feet, I knew I must have sustained serious damage because my legs began to jerk causing my body to fall backward onto the carpet. I managed to get to the phone, called my plumber, and explained what had happened. Thankfully, he called an ambulance that quickly arrived and got me to the hospital even before my plumber got to my house.

I was in the hospital for two weeks but had to stay off my feet for four months. My younger daughter, Susie, and her husband came to stay and help me out during this difficult recovery, and a home nurse came to change the bandages on my feet every day. Things like this happened all the time, but with the Lord's help, I overcame each one of them, one step at a time.

# A Message from God

My mother and I had many more opportunities to help and encourage each other when we lived together. We grew very close, and together we read through the entire Bible—a truly wonderful time for both of us. Our relationship with each other grew stronger as we shared many spiritual experiences together.

Once when my mother and I were attending one of the services at our church, a member of the congregation gave me a message that she said God had given to her through revelation that was meant for me (as follows):

> "Julia, my little lamb, I'm carrying you in my arms, and I will never let you go. Your ear is touching my chest. Can you hear my heart pounding its love for you? As you wake each day, remember that I'm holding you. We are together; we are never apart."
>
> "I have caught every tear you've cried. With each tear, we will water the earth and bring forth fruit for Father's garden. Let me show myself strong in your weakness. Let us offer sacrifice of praise. Exchange heaviness for the garment of praise."

"You are a royal princess in my kingdom. You have learned much already; I have much to show you still."

"Wait on me, worship me, lean on me. In spirit and truth you will magnify my word. You will be a tree of refreshment to the nations. Healing is in your leaves. Your light will draw many into my kingdom of life."

"Be anxious for nothing, for I am with you even until the end of the age. Arise, my daughter, and come away with me," says the Lord your God. Selah.

—Revelation given to me by church member

I received peace and comfort from such ministrations of the spirit. These messages were reinforcements for me that God had not abandoned me to my afflictions and that he did—and does—continue to love me.

Through my church affiliations, I met a man named Ollie who was involved with a prison ministry called Bridge Builders. Ollie and his members invited me to attend a prison ministry meeting with them one evening to share my spiritual testimony. When I told my story, the prisoners were inspired by my faith and endurance, and I believe I gave them hope too. I asked God to bless Ollie because of his great field work for the Lord. Each time I was privileged to share my testimony, I felt my own spirit grow stronger.

## The Lord Giveth (and Taketh Away)

Some of you may be familiar with the television evangelist Benny Hinn, best known for his healing ministry. I really enjoyed his ministry, and since he was scheduled to appear at a convention in North Carolina (not far from us), my daughter Donna arranged for me and my mother to attend. I was excited because I really felt that the Lord was going to touch me and my mother during the service, and he did.

One of the ushers approached me and said that God was healing me, and I absolutely rejoiced! I wanted my mother to be completely healed too, so I was praying intensely for her. The usher wanted to take me to the stage, but I wouldn't go because, for some reason, I was afraid to step out in public and show my faith by going up to the stage. But our God is so good, and he touched me anyway.

While all of us were getting back into the car to go home, I felt overcome with renewed strength. When we got back home, I started getting rid of my crutch and my medicines. For a while, my legs started working normally, and my insides did too. I was overjoyed, praying and thanking my Lord. I am not sure what happened, but I gradually started losing the healing following an incident that happened at the house causing fear to well up inside of me. I think I understand it now, but at that time, I did not.

I began to think about the time a pastor from another church I was attending told me that I did not have enough faith to walk without crutches. At the time, I thought, *What a thing for a man of God to say!* I was very hurt and resentful, but now I understand what the pastor meant. My Lord is teaching me so much that I could not have previously put into words. I just know that he has me in the palm of his hands.

It has also become clear to me that the Lord places people in our lives just when we need them the most. One such person was an old friend, Blanche, a former high school girlfriend of my older brother, Clyde, with whom I became reacquainted. We have gotten to be really good friends since meeting again. She is a very wonderful Christian lady with whom I have a great deal in common.

I thank God for the people in my life who give me constant love and encouragement; I've learned never to take any of the people in my life for granted.

Another life-changing event was about to occur when Don's sisters asked me to go with them to Medjugorje, Yugoslavia, on a pilgrimage to a famous holy site. I was told that when a couple went to Medjugorje together, they usually returned home more united because so many remarkable miracles and healings were taking place, in large numbers, at Medjugorje. So I asked Don to go with me, but he refused. Even though his refusal hurt, I decided to go anyway with my sisters-in-law.

## Medjugorje, Yugoslavia

Since 1981, when the original apparitions of the Virgin Mary reportedly appeared, many other apparitions followed manifesting in miraculous phenomena of all kinds, both in the sky and on the ground at Medjugorje (located in the former Yugoslavia). Scientists have tried to unravel the mystery surrounding the medically verified healings that have taken place in that renowned sacred place. There have been too many such stories to dismiss them as mere myth or hysterical hype.

Because I had nothing to lose and everything to gain, I knew I had to go there myself and find out if God had a message for me. I believed with all of my heart that I would come away with something that would help me understand the many "why" questions that filled my head after the accident and the loss of my marriage for a second time. I had never been angry with God over the things that happened to me, but there were times when I thought he might be angry with me. I had to know the truth.

Was there something I had done to incur the wrath of my beloved God? And, if so, I prayed that he would tell me.

My heart was full of repentance. I had suffered physical and emotional torments that had humbled me to the core of my being; I had suffered humiliation and losses that I would never understand in this lifetime.

Don's refusal to go with me only increased my determination to face God with all the humility that life had forced upon me. I needed answers.

## My Easter Sunday Miracle

I was in Medjugorje, Yugoslavia, on Easter Sunday, 1988. I had gone there expecting miracles because the Lord had already told me that he would be with me, and I believed it.

Most of the people in the different groups had gone up the mountain to the place where it was said the Holy Virgin had made herself visible to the faithful who were in need of her blessings. I saw that it would be a difficult walk for me even though I had dearly wanted to be up on the mountain with everyone else. As I turned, I saw a man standing behind me. I asked what he was doing, and he told me that he had come to help me get up the mountain. I thought this was unusual because I recognized him as the taxi driver who had driven us to the site from our hotel. With his help, I was able to join the others, and I felt very blessed to have had this kind man's assistance. I felt the spirit of the Lord with me, and I prayed fervently that he would bless me and let me feel his love.

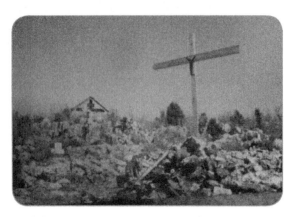

The sacred mountaintop at Medjugorje

After some time in prayer, I came down from the mountain and had just purchased some bottles to fill with holy water. When I entered the church courtyard, all of a sudden, I felt as though I had stepped into another dimension. I was immediately surrounded by all of the radiant colors of the rainbow and others I had never seen before, even more beautiful. The colors were pulsating as if they were alive and dancing.

Suddenly, I was embraced by a feeling of the most indescribable love. I also heard strains of beautiful, heavenly music that came from everywhere. I became engulfed in the brilliant colors and the music. As I looked around, I suddenly saw open fields of beautiful flowers swaying as though they were dancing. Then I saw hills and mountains so beautiful that I have no earthly words to describe them.

What followed was the most amazing part of my vision. I did not see the Lord, but I felt him, and I knew that it was Jesus who was embracing me with his wonderful arms and filling me with such indescribable peace; I never wanted it to end. Again, he told me that he loved me, that he would never leave me, and for me not to be afraid.

As suddenly as I had stepped into the vision, I stepped out of it. I stood for a moment reflecting on what had just happened to me and looked around to see where I was. The experience brought to my mind Paul's biblical vision when he said, "I did not know if I was in the third heaven."

I was still so much in a trance from what had just happened that when I looked around and saw a statue where people were praying, I didn't know if I was still on earth or had been transported somewhere else. I just knew that the Lord had allowed me to experience a little bit of heaven, and I did not want it to end. I looked around to see whether anyone else was experiencing something unusual, but everyone seemed to be acting quite normal. For me, it was as if time had just stood still, or as though there was no such thing as the concept of time; it was amazing!

I truly have no words to describe, with my earthly vocabulary, the entire vision, but I do know now that I *know, know, know* that God *is* real and that his heaven *is* real!

After I had settled my thoughts back to earth, I proceeded to the fountain by the church to fill up my bottles with holy water. When I turned to enter the church, I saw that it was encased in the most magnificent rainbow of colors.

*Oh my!* This was truly a miracle that I will never forget. I went into the church and prayed. I was overcome with the spirit of pure love; I just wanted to stay in the church and never come out. It was about midnight when I finally went outside. Apparently my sisters-in-law had been looking all over for me.

"There you are!," they said with concerned expressions on their faces.

I told the ladies that they should have known I would be inside the church; they laughed when they realized it was the first place they should have searched for me.

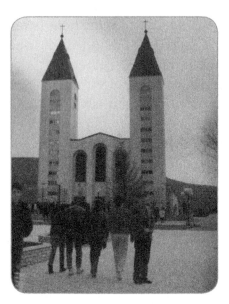

The church at Medjugorje

As my group stood talking, I looked up and saw a man standing at the corner of the church who began walking toward us with his eyes focused directly on me. As he approached, he handed me a picture and told me that the Lord wanted me to have it. I felt so blessed, and my sisters-in-law asked, "What did he give you?" I showed them the picture of Mary and the Christ child that I have kept to this day. I truly believe that the unknown man was also an angel who had come to comfort me with something I could keep as a remembrance of my miracle Easter Sunday in Medjugorje.

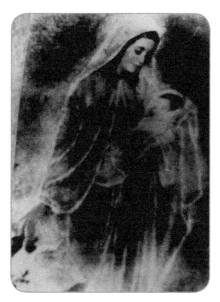

The picture I was given of the
Virgin Mary and Christ child

## On Fire for the Lord

When my sisters-in-law and I returned to the states from Medjugorje, I was so full of the spirit of the Lord that my husband called me a fanatic. I said, "No, I'm not, I just love my Lord." There was no way for Don to understand the things that I told him about the miracle I had witnessed there.

My spirit had been touched in ways that there are simply no words to describe. I have learned that when a person receives a personal revelation from the Lord, it is almost indefinable with mortal language because he communicates with us in the language of pure spirit.

It was during this time that I stopped going to the Catholic church and started attending a full gospel, nondenominational church where I felt the Lord had led me. I have no ill will against the Catholic church and do not wish to give that impression; I simply found a way that seems to better express my own spiritual feelings.

While I was going to a full gospel church, one Wednesday evening service, I received a vision. I saw an open space where a table was surrounded by twelve elders who sat ensconced in a halo of brilliant lights. That was all I saw in the vision.

I had another vision at the same full gospel church during the evening service in March 1995. As the choir sang, the Lord showed me an awe-inspiring vision wherein I saw the people of our congregation standing at the foot of the cross looking up at Jesus, the Lamb of God, who had sacrificed himself for us all. As we were beholding the Lamb of God on the cross, he suddenly began ascending toward heaven encircled by radiating, brilliant light. As he arose, he gathered all of us close around him and held us tightly within the brilliant light that engulfed and became him. We too became immersed into this pure, refulgent light and began to arise toward heaven with him. The light had become more and more brilliant and radiant as we ascended. Although we were traveling at a very high speed, we experienced a sense of wonderful peace and well-being bathed in the light of Christ. We continued to rise with him until we came into the heavenly kingdom where there appeared to be beautiful crystals everywhere. Jesus then lowered us down in front of him. We were all bowing with arms outstretched toward him in praise. He became even more brilliant and radiant with his arms outstretched, with unconditional love toward us. He wore a beautiful golden crown around his head signifying the power of his holy lineage, and within that indescribably beautiful light, we felt the loving omniscience of our Creator God so powerfully that we did not want it to stop. The brilliance and intensity of the light was hard to behold, but it did not hurt our eyes. After some time with Jesus, he began gently pushing us back toward the earth accompanied by the force of his brilliant light. Then I saw that each of us had a beautiful crown placed upon our own heads. I did not know at the time what exactly this vision meant, but the Lord kept telling me to share the vision until I heard one of the associate pastors say something about the anointing. It was then that the Spirit brought the meaning of the vision into my mind, which was that God had placed his special golden anointing upon us all. Praise God forevermore. Amen.

As I tried to give witness of the Lord's healing powers to others and shared the details of my own story, it became apparent that they had difficulty believing me because I *looked* normal and they just could not see how truly handicapped I was. Even the doctors had difficulty with this, until they saw my records. When any doctor saw my medical history, many would say that I was a true miracle.

During one of my many doctor's appointments, Dr. Young wanted to go over some of the MRIs that had just been completed. When I was in his office, he had placed my x-rays on the wall-mounted light box for viewing but asked me to wait just a moment.

He called some of the interns into his office because he was also an instructing physician. As they filed in, Dr. Young asked the interns to look at my x-rays on the viewer. After they had all seen the x-rays, he then asked me to stand up.

When I did as he asked, Dr. Young told the interns to look at the x-rays again then to look at me. He said that according to the x-rays, I should not be standing, much less walking. He called me a miracle and said that I "was walking only by the grace of God." I told him that I knew this as fact.

I had a lot of prophecies given to me while I was going to the various churches during the time I lived with my mother.

My mother had been suffering from complications of long-term diabetes and had been hospitalized and scheduled for amputation of a gangrenous limb. All of my brothers and sisters helped out; every one of us did as much as we could do to encourage, call, and visit her as often as possible. I have to say that I have some wonderful brothers and sisters who would go out of their way to help anyone in need. They were always encouraging and supportive to me and my mother; I love them all dearly.

## A Peaceful Passing

On the morning of the day my mother passed on to heaven, I woke up and went to the bathroom where my sister Connie was getting ready for work. By that time, she had moved in with mother and me, and it was wonderful to have her there with us. I wished Connie a good morning then went back to bed and fell asleep. When I awoke, I saw that Connie was still getting ready for work, which was strange because it seemed like ages since I had gone back to sleep, but it must only have been a few minutes between falling asleep and awaking the second time. I told Connie that I had just received an amazing vision and began describing it to her.

In the vision, I had seen a beautiful home, but outside, there were two huge, ominous animals—an elephant and a gorilla—trying to storm down the front door. I invoked the name of Jesus, and in his holy name, I bound the invading animals against any harm to those who were inside. In the next scene, I was standing in a room and looking outside through a huge picture window where I saw beautiful scenery with all kinds of animals playing peacefully; it was so beautiful, and the colors were indescribable. I was overcome with such a feeling of peacefulness! Then I turned my attention back inside the house and saw my mother in the dining room of the home where we had been living. She was radiant and looked as young as she had during her thirties, with long black hair, a beautiful figure, and she was happily swirling around in a gleeful dance. I then noticed my father in the kitchen sitting in a rocking chair with a slight smile on his face.

When I finished telling my sister about the vision, she felt prompted to go to the hospital to visit my mother. I talked to Momma on the phone several times that day but could not go see her because I had taken some pills, which kept me home. I was still paralyzed internally with no feelings from my chest down and could not use my left hand, but I always managed with the Lord's help using one crutch to get around after the total knee replacement had been performed on my left leg.

Connie went to the hospital that evening to visit Momma and to feed her supper. During this time, Momma asked Connie, "What are all those little white snowflakes floating around everywhere?"

Connie said that she didn't know, but when she told me about it, I said, "Oh, Connie, those were the angels coming for her."

That night, Momma went on to heaven. I was very sad as were all of my brothers and sisters. I asked the Lord to give me some kind of sign that I might know my dear mother was all right. I was restless around midnight and got out of bed and went into Momma's room. Right outside her bedroom window, I heard the most beautiful music coming from a little bird. I knew that my mother was with our Lord and that she was happy.

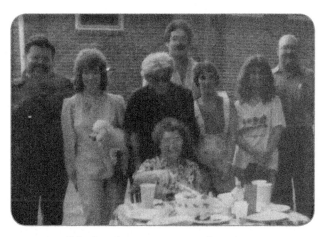

My brothers, sisters, and parents
*Back left,* Gary; *back right,* David; *middle from left to right,* Clyde, me, Dad, Sherry, and Connie; *front,* Mom

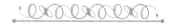

# A New Career?

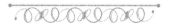

After my mother had died, I went to live in Gloucester, Virginia, where the doctors sent me to the Disability Rehabilitation Center, close to Waynesboro, Virginia, where I could learn a skill that would enable me to get a job doing something useful given the conditions of my handicap. I had always loved reading, so I chose to become a librarian. It was a lot of hard work since I had not been to school for quite some time, but I was thrilled when I finally received my degree of which I was really proud. When I tried to get a job at the library, however, those in charge of hiring told me that I was too handicapped for such a position. This rejection made me feel useless for a while, especially after working so hard to obtain my education. But again, I looked on the bright side of things and was happy about living by myself and having my own home again.

During this time, my younger daughter Susie and her family came home from Russia where they had been missionaries and moved in with me until they got back on their feet financially. Her husband found a job as a plumber in Richmond after about five months, so they left for Richmond to live there. I was so grateful that I had a place for them to stay.

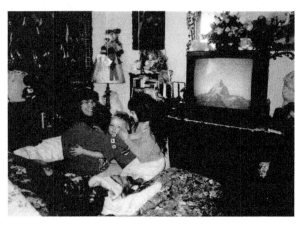

Me and my darling grandchildren, Elisha and Gabriel

## The Wedding Present

When Don and I first got married in 1956, the first thing that we bought for each other was our family Bible. He also had gotten me a crucifix/cross necklace for a wedding present. I really loved it and wore it all the time, never taking it off for anything or any reason.

One morning while I was cleaning the bathroom at my home in Gloucester (after Don had left me for the second time), leaning over the toilet and then flushing it, I noticed that my cross had fallen off the chain into the toilet bowl and was flushed away before I could react. This was the one place that I could not retrieve it. I was very upset about losing it, and it occurred to me that this was forty years to the date when Don had originally given me the cross. Losing the cross felt as though God was telling me to let go of the past. I also realized that God wanted me to know I should never have anything that I cherish above him—significant moment of truth that I have never forgotten.

Since I had not been permitted to work as a librarian, I took several jobs during this time, one of which was as a driver of a handicapped bus. I managed well with God's and my children's help. It was also during this year that I wrote a letter to the actor Christopher Reeve (known for his wonderful portrayal of the comic book hero *Superman*), but I didn't mail it. When I finally decided to send the letter, I found out that Mr. Reeve had died. This was a very sad occasion for everyone, but I know that he is happy now in heaven with our Lord. Below is an insert of the letter that I had written to him addressed to his wife.

## The Letter I Never Sent

March 28, 1997
Dear Mrs. Reeves:

I wrote this letter to your husband to hopefully encourage and help him to realize that all things are possible—just never give up. Keep a positive outlook always. Instead of sending the letter to your husband, Christopher, I decided to send it to you so that you could read it and decide if it would be encouraging to him. I pray for him and you. This is a very difficult period you are going through right now (I know; I've been there), but I just know you are going to pull through this, and it will make you both closer than you have ever been.

    I watched you on the show *20/20*, and I got the feeling that you are a very strong woman and that your love has made a wonderful union between you and your husband. I praise the Lord for this.

    I wrote this letter not long after your husband's accident, but I've taken so long in sending it because I have been very sick. I hope and pray now is a good time to send this letter, with the enclosed articles, and that my struggle in overcoming will be an inspiration to both of you. You are a wonderful woman and person.

Keep strong and pray with one another. That is very important.

God Bless You,<br>Julia Widlacki

P.S. I do hope to meet you both.

Dear Christopher,

I feel as if I know you already, but I realize that I don't. I suppose that when people are famous, everyone has the feeling of knowing that person and feel a closeness to him or her.

My heart goes out to you, Christopher, because I truly know what you are going through. But with the Lord's help and your inner strength that He gives all of us, you will pull through even this. You will be an overcomer. I always think that way—always think positive—even though things seem to be at their darkest. God promised us that He would never leave or forsake us, and it seems to me that you have a very positive outlook on life, so that's half the battle already won.

I am a walking quadriplegic—that is how the medical community classifies my condition—which means that I am a quadriplegic, but I can walk; I praise the Lord for this. I broke my neck in a car accident in 1967 when I was twenty-seven years old and married with five little children. My youngest at the time was five years old. It was very hard on my husband and children because I stayed in the hospital for almost a year. My doctor told my husband not to expect me to walk again, but I was a very determined person. I have always had a positive outlook on life and a strong belief in God. I know that with God, everything is possible.

After the accident, I was taken to the hospital where they operated on my neck and put tongs in my head. When I woke up and came to my senses, so to speak, I was lying in a bed, unable to move, and it felt like my whole body (insides) were on fire. It was difficult to breathe, and the internal pain seemed too much to bear. I had forty-five pounds of weight keeping my head from moving and to keep the pressure off my spine. The doctors operated to remove bone fragments, as they did with you.

I broke my neck at the C5, C6, and C7 vertebrae, and that has left me paralyzed from the neck down. I realize that your neck is broken higher up, so it is affecting your breathing, but hang in there; it will get better. Be careful not to move your head, and do everything that the medical staff suggests. You are in good hands. That's the one thing I have to say about my recovery; I had excellent doctors.

After the accident, I lay in Intensive Care for fifteen days, and since I couldn't do anything, I just concentrated on moving my big toe. I would just lie there with my eyes closed and told my brain to tell my toe to move. And, on the fifteenth day, my toed moved! Everyone jumped for joy. I was then taken out of the Intensive Care Unit placed in a special circular bed, and there I remained for four months. I would be placed on my back for two hours, then on my stomach for two hours, and I would keep concentrating on moving different parts of my body. I could eventually move my arms, but not my hands. My husband came to the hospital twice a day to feed me, and I know this was very hard on him.

I am not saying that I never got down, but when I did, I would quickly think positive thoughts. I dreamed a lot of dreams during that time, things that I would do when I got better.

After the doctors removed the tongs from my head, they put a steel neck brace on me and let me sit in a wheelchair. I was finally able to see my children, which was wonderful because I hadn't seen them during the four months that I was in special care. After this, I began therapy. I was placed on a tilt table, and every time they did this, I asked them to unstrap me because I knew that I could walk. In my own mind, I could do this, but when they finally allowed me to try, I collapsed (haha!) but kept my faith and kept telling myself, "I can walk, I can do this!"

Again, after some time, the therapists unstrapped me again, and I took one step and passed out over the therapist's shoulder and woke up in bed. But I did it! I kept progressing on from there. Everyone at the hospital began calling me their miracle girl. Each time one of the staff came to weigh me, I would insist that they allow me to stand. Every time that they acquiesced, I would pass out on them—but I was progressing, and I was very happy about that!

Eventually I was allowed to come home and was forced to face a whole new life situation. My husband was wonderful and never complained, but I felt terrible because I was such a burden.

In about two years, I was able to walk without a walker or a cane, and it felt incredible! Each triumph was a marvel. I was still unable to use my hands, and I was still paralyzed internally with no feelings in my body from my chest down, but I did everything I could do to look normal. I would even walk to the beauty shop to have my hair washed and often pushed beyond my limits just to prove that I could do things that took some of the pressure off my husband, Don, who also made some amazing gadgets that helped me perform tasks I would otherwise not have been able to do.

I was progressing very well until 1976 when I had another car accident and smashed my left knee that required me to have an entire knee replacement.

Through three operations and six more months in the hospital, I was back in a wheelchair again, with a brace on my left leg. But I was not beaten! I did everything I could do to walk again. This time, however, I was not able to do away with the crutches, but I now need only one to help me walk. I had lost ground, but I was still able to keep going.

The second accident really took its toll on my husband, and even though he really gave of himself, the conditions of my ongoing dependence got the best of him, and after thirty years of marriage, he felt cheated out of life because of having to care for a handicapped wife. I will always love him because he was a wonderful man and husband. I sometimes believe that it is harder on the healthier person than it is on the injured one who has gotten hurt and has no choice. In the final analysis, it's the healthy spouse who has to make some of the difficult decisions in order to retain their own sanity.

During this time, there was no one we knew who could counsel with us and help us with our unique situation. My advice is to find someone with whom you can communicate. It is very important to have someone trained to help, especially when there is a family involved. Since Don and I did not have such help, I don't blame him for his decision to leave; I only wish him well. He is now remarried and seems to have a very nice wife. I ask God's blessing on them and just hope one day that my ex-husband and I will be able to have a friendly relationship. But honestly, it really devastated me. The feeling of such a rejection by someone you love so deeply is almost more than one can bear.

I must add that after Don and I were divorced, I continued to try and win him back from his girlfriend at the time, and somehow it worked. Don and I were remarried to each other, but it lasted only one month. I could see that Don tried, but after that month, he again asked for a divorce, which hurt me even more than it did the first time and possibly even more than the devastation of the accident.

I have tried to pick up the pieces of my life since then, but it has been a struggle. With God's help, though, I am making it day by day. I will be victorious in Jesus' name, and you will be too. Believe that, because you have what it takes, and you are God's child.

Love in Christ Jesus,<br>Julia Widlacki

I wrote much more in my letter to Christopher Reeve but have elected to share only the portion above, because much of my story has already been shared with my readers. I have a single regret about this letter—that I did not send it after I had felt inspired to write it. Another lesson learned—we should never procrastinate doing the things we feel inspired to do.

## Life on My Own

During the time I lived alone in my house, I fell several times, and due to certain injuries I had sustained, I required another total knee replacement. It was during this time that I had to have the surgery for my right leg where the doctors performing the repair had cut an artery, and I almost bled to death. Had God not intervened through my oldest daughter Donna and the vascular surgeon whom was not supposed to be there that day, I would have died. The orthopedic doctor who did the knee surgery was so thankful that I was caught in time, that he gave me a hug and said, "Julia, you have angels watching over you."

My sister-in-law, Judy, kept in touch with me quite often. We shared the same birthday. The following is a message from the card Judy sent me on my birthday that illustrates her kindness toward me.

Julia, my dear, dear friend:

You call me the most precious lady in all the world, but you already hold that title, and I don't presume that I am as precious and special as you are. Julia, you're going to have to promise to pull me up to the mansion God has prepared for me. I kind of hope that we'll be neighbors, but I'm probably on the wrong side of the tracks from where you'll be. But praise God, He won't allow me to feel the difference. I will be as happy as I can possibly be. You have suffered so much and have cheerfully offered your sufferings to our Good Shepherd so that He can take care of all of His lambs. Julia, maybe someday you will understand the esteem and love that I have for you, but you are so humble, and I probably won't see that day until much later. My dear sister and good friend, I love you, respect you, and thank God for letting me know you.

Judy

Judy has always been a source of encouragement and hope to me. She is a wonderful lady along with her sister Mickey. I pray God's blessings on all of them forever.

# Time for a Change

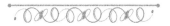

When my youngest daughter, Susie, came down to visit me, she observed that I could no longer live by myself because I kept falling and that I needed to live with one of my children. My older daughter, Donna, who lived nearby, always came over and helped me a great deal but was unable to take me in due to circumstances beyond her control. My youngest daughter, Susie, and her husband volunteered to take me into their home, so I moved in with them in Richmond. She and her husband were ministers, and she also homeschooled her six children. Aside from being a minister of the gospel, Susie's husband became a master plumber. It was a very lively, busy household of which I enjoyed being a part. I was in and out of the hospital a lot with additional surgeries while I lived with them. Not only were they a great help to me, but she and her husband helped me to grow in the Lord. I loved living with my younger daughter and her family; they are truly an amazing family.

After six years of staying with my youngest daughter, my youngest son, Guy, had called me and asked if I would be willing to come live with him and his two children because his wife had abandoned them, and he wanted me to be there as a loving motherly support. I said yes, I would love to stay with him and his children if they needed me. My youngest son, Guy, now takes care of me, along with his two beautiful children and the help of all my other children—Donna, Donny, Tim, and Susie. I also receive help from nurses and home health aides and would especially like to mention Rosie and Serita who have been a constant blessing to me.

I go to my son's church in Portsmouth, Virginia, as I am able, and our pastor and his wife have been and continue to be an inspiration to me. I thank them for their guidance, support, and prayers.

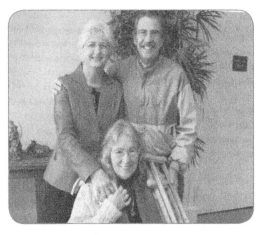

In a recent picture, *left back row,* Pastor Keith's wife, Pat; *right back row,* Pastor Keith Lewis; *front row,* me

I have had many additional surgeries and hospitalizations since 2003, but the Lord has led and guided me every step of the way. In August 2011, he prompted my spirit with the following scripture:

> Remember how the Lord your God led you on this long journey through the desert these past 40 years sending hardships to test you so that He might know what you intended to do and whether you would obey His commands. He made you go hungry and

then He gave you manna to eat, food that you and your ancestors have never eaten before. He did this to teach you that man must not depend on bread alone to sustain him but on everything that the Lord says.

During these 40 years, your clothes have not worn out(and mine haven't) nor have your feet swollen up. Remember that the Lord your God corrects and punishes you just as a father disciplines his children.

So then, do as the Lord has commanded you. Live according to His laws and obey Him. The Lord your God is bringing you into a fertile land, a land that has rivers and springs, and underground streams gushing out into the valleys and hills, a land that produces wheat and barley, grapes, figs, pomegranates, olives and honey. There you will never go hungry or ever be in need. Its rocks have iron in them, and from its hills you can mine copper.

You will have all you want to eat and you will give thanks to the Lord your God for the fertile land that He has given you.

Deuteronomy 8:2–10<br>(St. Jerome Catholic Study Bible)

I found this scripture to be especially relevant because forty years had passed since my accident.

## Understanding God's Messages

Over the years, so many people have asked me, "If you have such belief and faith in God, why are you not completely healed and are not walking with total healing?" I say to these people that I know I am healed; God has already healed me. Why it has not manifested yet in the natural, I go to 2 Corinthians 12:7–10:

> But to keep me from being puffed up with pride, because of the many wonderful things I saw, I was given a painful, physical ailment, which acts as

Satan's messenger, to beat me and keep me from being proud. Three times I prayed to the Lord about this and asked Him to take it away, but His answer was, "My grace is all you need, for my power is greatest when you are weak." I am most happy then to be proud of my weaknesses in order to feel the protection of Christ's power over me. I am content with weaknesses, insults, hardships, persecutions and difficulties for Christ's sake...for when I am weak then I am strong.

(Reference: St. Jerome Catholic Study Bible)

I will, therefore, always give praises to my God, my Lord and Savior, Jesus Christ. He said that he would always be with me and never leave me. I honor and praise him forever for the constant care and understanding that he has continued to provide.

I want to add here that we need always to forgive others so that our prayers will not be hindered and so the Lord will forgive us.

We are promised that as we forgive, we also will be forgiven.

## Looking Back

I look back now and see that I have truly been taking one step at a time, overcoming one obstacle at a time, just like my Lord had told me to do in a vision where I looked up at him as his arms were outstretched to me with his holy angels ascending up one side and descending down the other of a beautiful golden stairway saying, "Don't be afraid, my daughter, I am always with you. I love you."

I am so grateful that my Father has given me this vision and a *knowing* that I have been growing in him, one step at a time. I cannot wait to take the stair steps to heaven of which my Lord has given me a preview from one glory realm to the next; from one "maturity" level to the next.

# My Loving Family: Their Stories

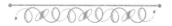

We never know the real influence we have over other people, how they view us, or what our real impact has been when measured over a lifetime. We are always being observed by someone, and I have always prayed that my influence has been a good one.

Two of my grandchildren have written their individual tributes to me that have touched my heart so deeply that I wish to reprint them for my readers.

I don't include these personal stories and poems for the sake of enhancing my own ego but to pay a returned tribute to these dear ones who have given me so much love and support that I would feel greatly remiss if I didn't include them in my book. Following is a school essay that my grandson Gabriel wrote. Although he was quite serious about the title, I have to admit it made me smile.

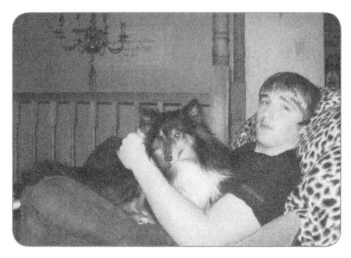

My grandson Gabriel Bane

## My Long-Suffering Grandmother

(Reprinted as originally written)
By Gabriel Bane

My grandmother became an example of a longsuffering person, who despite all of her circumstances, never gives up her will to live.

My grandmother was in an automobile accident at the age of twenty-seven. Two drunk teens ran a stoplight and T-boned my grandmother's car. Her neck was broken in the accident. She has been a quadriplegic ever since, with an average lifespan of ten years. This prognosis did not stop my grandmother's will to walk. It has been forty-five years since the accident and she is still walking with the use of only crutches. Her eyes show small laugh lines coming from their edges.

The doctors said she would never walk again. (She does, though) Her faith in God, in the face of adversity, is memorable. She has endured so much; I cannot even begin to comprehend how much—yet, through it all, she keeps a smile on her face, a positive attitude on life, and hope in a future with Christ.

Now, she is not just a crippled grandmother that we all love and envy, no, she is an example of the Biblical concept of a woman of longsuffering with long enduring hope and joy. She has never lost her love for others. Even people outside of our family see her as a strong, loving person. I definitely cannot believe that through all this, she forgave those two guys that caused this continuous suffering.

Guess what she says, almost all of the time? "Praise the Lord in all things." Her eyes continue to glisten in the sunlight and her face shines as someone who knows of a hope not yet to come. Her hair is whitening with age as her body degrades, yet, in all this, my grandmother is an incredible human being that we could all learn a lesson or two from.

The following poem written by my grandson Michael Hepner was published in *The International Who's Who in Poetry*, an anthology compiled by the International Library of Poetry.

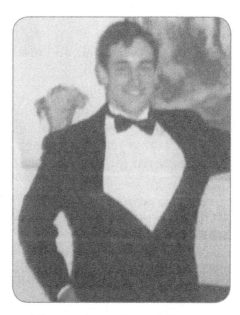

My grandson Michael Hepner

*Julia Dean Childress Widlacki*

## Purpose

By Michael Hepner

There comes a time
In the lives of many
When our purpose is revealed

To each their own
A passion for being
A thing to call their dream

Many are called, few are chosen
The work at hand is great

You touch the lives of many
Even when you are away
Your memory shall never fade in their hearts

God made you special
A jewel in the eyes of the Lord
A light for all to see

Loving, long-suffering, tranquil, and meek
All who meet you sneak a peak
At the light from your mystique

Thank you, Grandma, for your love,
I shall never forget your purpose for me,
The light you imparted for all to see

My daughter Susan also wrote me a poem on Valentine's Day of 2014. I thought I would add this along with my grandson's poem. It is entitled *Mama*.

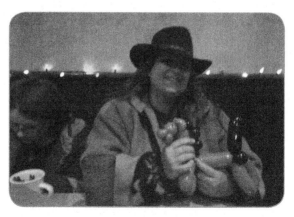

My daughter Susan Bane

## Mama

You have been an inspiration to me throughout my life
You have been a light that shines bright
Your courage & perseverance staggers me
I have learned these traits by watching you
Your love of life is incredible
Your love of all things living is inspiring
Your life of prayer is a lesson to me
I have learned these traits by watching you
The late night talks are such a blessing to me
Your love of Jesus Christ is an anchor to me
Your devotion to what is true and honest are lights for me
I have learned these traits by watching you
Your ability to move beyond the natural is incredible to me
Your ability to see all things good means more than life to me
Your insight to things I have yet to understand is so worth searching out to me
Your wisdom, kindness, gentleness, & love are everything to me!
I have learned these traits by watching you

I love you Mama more than all the stars in the sky
Surrounded by rainbows of infinite beauty!

Love forever,<br>Sue, your daughter

The following is a poem that was written by my lovely mother, and the truth of her words touches my heart.

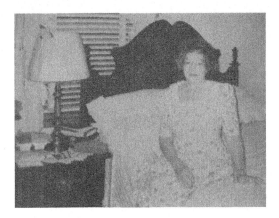

My mother, Margaret McCall Childress

### Reach for a Star

By Margaret McCall Childress

Time is swiftly passing by
As we live each day a new.
We reach for heights undreamed of
But the heights we reach are few
So strive for great achievements
And be a better man by far
What can we be, but failures
If we don't reach for a star.

T'was the drive man put behind him
That gave us a merry tune
That same great drive in motion
Flew a rocket to the moon

Think big, think great thoughts always
For thoughts materialize
Never think small, just dream a good dream
And that dream you'll realize.
So, strive for greater achievements
And be a better man by far
What can we be, but failures
If we don't reach for a star.

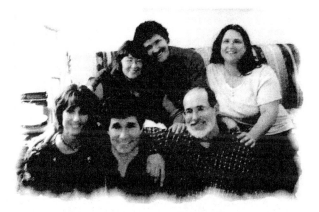

Me and my beautiful children
*Back row, left to right,* Julia Dean, Tim, and Susan;
*front row, left to right,* Donna, Guy, and Donny

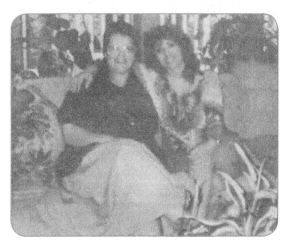

My lovely daughters, Sue and Donna

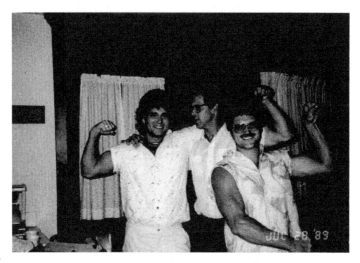

My three handsome sons, 1989
*Left to right:* Guy, Donny, and Tim

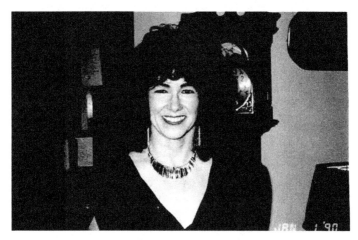

Me, January 1990

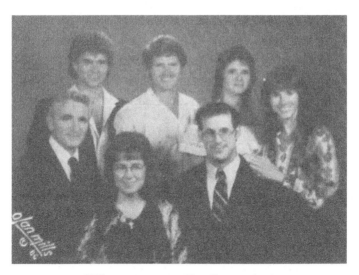

When we were all still together
*Back row, left to right,* Guy, Tim, Sue, and Donna;
*front row, left to right,* Don, me, and Donny

## They Were All Victims…

My grown children and I recently sat around my brother Clyde's dining room table discussing the impact that my accident and subsequent handicap had on my children while I was still in the hospital and when I returned home after a year of convalescence.

I was surprised to hear that Donny and Tim said that they had blocked out many childhood memories. Sue's memories began to pick up during a brief time in therapy when she was able to recall details of our family life when Don was away in Vietnam in 1970. Tim said, "There are things in our lives that we try not to remember because they are just too painful." Donna however was simply unable to remember certain events possibly because she had sustained three concussions to include the one sustained in the family car accident.

I think my children have now begun to realize, as I have, that facing painful memories, though initially disturbing to one's peace of mind, is the only road to healing.

Following are the stories from each of my five children detailing their memories and physical/emotional "traumas" they experienced during their childhood and throughout their adult lives. As you read their stories, you will see how God's hand has truly protected my entire family, and I cannot thank him enough.

## Sue Remembers

Just before I had left the house on the day of my devastating car accident, my six-year-old daughter, Susie, and I had been having an argument about something that I can't recall, but Sue remembers it as the usual contest of wills that, according to her, she always lost. Even at six years old, Susie was quite rebellious when it came to being told what to do; therefore, it's quite possible that our argument had been about chores that she didn't want to do or didn't think was fair (to her). I had no idea of the degree of anger that my young daughter had felt for me on that day that caused her such emotional damage until many years later.

For some reason that wasn't clear to me, Sue and my relationship always seemed strained and distant, and her attitude toward me lasted for many years, well into her adulthood. I knew that she loved me, but there seemed to be a wall between us that neither of us could breach.

Sue had gone through many trials during her childhood and young adulthood years, but we were not very close in ways that she felt she could confide in me. Some of the trials I will not mention for the sake of, and respect for, Sue's privacy. I have my daughter's permission to discuss one of the most significant events that eventually helped me to understand her withdrawal on an emotional level that kept us from sharing the most natural love between mother and daughter. Happily, I can report that we are able to enjoy a renewed loving relationship, in full measure, at this time.

## Sue's Story (in Her Words)

As I grew up, I was a great deal like my father and preferred the company of Dad and my brothers to that of my sister and mother. I liked to be outside and spent a great deal of time with Dad and the boys. I prided myself in being a tomboy, not a girly-girl who stayed inside and did "women's work." My sister Donna had grown to accept that role, and she helped mom so much that I can't even imagine how my mother would have survived without Donna.

I could tell that my mother found it difficult to understand some of my choices; she knew that I had experimented with drugs and alcohol. She saw that I was seeking my own path in places she did not approve, but because of our strained relationship, she had little influence over me. I know my mother watched with a broken heart, but she knew, as all parents do, that I would have to find my own way. She didn't nag, but I remember the hurt in her eyes wondering when I would come to my senses. Any criticism from her would have only made things worse, so she prayed for my safety and that my heart would turn to the Lord during my search for life's greatest answers and inner peace.

I married as soon as I was eighteen, and after suffering many trials, I finally gave my life to the Lord, and later, my husband and I were sent by our church to Russia on an evangelical mission trip for ten and a half months. After our mission was completed, we returned home and moved in with my mom. We stayed with her for five months while we were getting back on our feet.

Even though we lived together, I still felt there was something unresolved between us, and I remember feeling strangely distant and uncomfortable when my mother gave me a hug or kissed my cheek.

From as far back as I could remember, Mother would pray over each of us at bedtime, a prayer that she still prays over us today. She would place her thumb on our foreheads and make the sign of the cross as she prayed, "May the Almighty God, Father, Son, and Holy Spirit bless you, my child, now and for eternity, and may this blessing remain with you forever, in Jesus' name, amen." She would kiss us, told us that she loved us, and wished us a good night and sweet dreams.

The prayer had always been a sweet reminder of my mother's love, but even when she prayed for me, I still felt a chasm between us. Something was definitely wrong!

One day at church, while we were still living with Mama, my pastor said something that pricked my heart because it was something I recognized deep inside that I hadn't admitted but would eventually have to face. He told me quietly, in my ear, that I had to "make things right with someone in my life." I knew immediately that it was my mother. We had such a strained relationship, yet I wanted to love her. I didn't understand what was stopping me from showing her the true affection of a daughter, so I prayed and asked the Lord what I should do.

I asked him to help me love my mother without animosity and without any hesitation in my heart.

I heard the Lord speak so clearly to me in these words: "I want you to serve your mother breakfast in bed for four weeks, placing a rose on her tray, and you are to sit with her the entire time."

All I could think was, *Wow! Okay.*

So on the way home from church, I bought a fabric rose, and the next morning I began to do exactly what the Lord told me to do. At first I didn't know what to do as I sat stiffly on the edge of her bed. Our conversations were strained, but after three or four days, our talks became easier and more substantive. I also began to remember things, private things, that I began to confess. I began to recall the events and feelings that had caused me to withdraw from her.

I remembered having been furious with her on the day of her accident, and *God help me,* I had actually wished she was dead. After her accident, I was certain that my hateful wish had come true and that I alone was responsible for what had happened to my mother. That terrible guilt followed me like a millstone around my neck. I became unable to respond to my mother because I needed to block out everything that was associated with what happened to her that I believed was my doing alone. The only way to fix what was wrong between us required me to be completely honest, and it was not easy!

### The Hard Stuff...

Mom's parents came out to our house to help our family before Mom was released from the hospital. We had gone through several house sitters, and I know that Dad didn't know what to do anymore with all of his added responsibilities and so little help.

It was during this time when my grandparents were staying with us, in Kansas, for a couple of months, that my grandfather (Mom's dad) began to molest me. I was only six years old, and because I had already blamed myself for Mom's accident, I also took the added blame for my grandfather's actions upon myself. I felt abandoned and helpless, and Mom wasn't there to help me.

After she got out of the hospital, our family moved to Virginia to be closer to her parents. During the drive there, I tried to kill myself by opening the side door and falling out of the car. Dad saw me and grabbed my shirt as I was falling; he kept me from completing my first suicide attempt.

I didn't want to move anywhere close to my grandfather. I was so frightened that I shut down deep inside myself since I couldn't tell anyone what was happening. I continued the habit of blaming myself for everything bad that happened to me after Mom's accident. After our move to Virginia, almost every time we went to my grandfather's house, for the next four years, he would find occasions to sexually molest me. For a long time, I had blocked out most of it, and I believe my grandfather's molestation stopped only because we didn't visit him after Dad went to Vietnam for a year. That was one of the best years of my entire childhood; it was such a peaceful time with just us kids, alone with our mother.

When I was fourteen, my dad told me to come into his bedroom to do things of which I would rather not speak of at this time. He also came into my room, and I begged him not to do anything like that again with me. He actually left my room, and thankfully, that part of my relationship with my father ended.

Then when I was fifteen, Dad told me that he wanted to divorce Mom and marry me! I was so shocked and confused so much so that I only stood there. I don't exactly remember what happened right after that, but I did go to my mother and told her what was happening. After confiding in my mother, Dad totally stopped approaching me. This was the first time that I ever talked to Mom about anything important in my life, and she shared with me some of the awful things that had happened to her at the hands of her father. Even though Mom was willing to help me with this, I still felt no close bond with her. My dark feelings ran deep, and they continued to fester as I grew older.

I remember another time when I was fifteen that our family was traveling together in our car when I yelled at Mom and told her that I hated her. Dad turned around and smacked me. As a kid, I didn't realize how much I was hurting her; I just didn't know how to connect with anyone on an intimate level. I only knew that I was hurting and felt alone and abandoned.

I was almost raped by a man when I was sixteen, but I managed to escape. When I ran into the house and told my Dad about it, he just ignored it, and so did everyone else. Everyone acted as though it had never happened—just one more thing that I held against my mother. She should have taken my side; someone should have!

I was sixteen when I went into the hospital to have my tonsils removed, and after the surgery, I got an infection that caused me to remain there for several days. My father would not allow anyone to visit me because I had not gone to see my mother in the hospital after her last accident. Dad dropped me off and picked me up. I felt so isolated and so very lonely, which, to my mind, provided more justification for the hostility I felt toward my mother. At that time of my life, she seemed to be at the core of every bad thing that happened to me and to my family.

Things were going downhill very rapidly in my young life. When I was seventeen, Dad had me admitted to the psychiatric unit of the hospital because I had wanted to kill myself. Even though I had been subjected to all kinds of questions about why I felt suicidal, I told the doctors nothing. Dad again would not allow anyone to visit me because I had refused to see my mother during her stays in the hospital. I was in the psych unit all alone for a solid week.

I had grown to harbor way too much anger, regret, and guilt, and my emotions were causing havoc in every aspect of my life.

Guilt is a powerful emotion and one that's not easily abandoned after a lifetime of feeling responsible for the hurt caused by oneself to another. I had finally faced my guilt and shared my deepest emotions with my mother; she in turn shared hers with me. The emotional flood banks overflowed as we sat each morning over breakfast revealing the hidden emotions and secrets that nearly destroyed me. We talked of my childhood and how I felt the need for a mom like the other little girls that I knew had. I told her of the disappointments I had felt when she wasn't there for me. I also told her about all of the blame I had placed on myself, and oddly (to me), my mother confessed that *she* felt responsible for all of the hardships that I had endured after her accident.

We embraced and cried a lot that day and several days to come. Sharing our true feelings became the salve to our wounded souls that enabled a great healing to take place. We were both able to clearly see that the accident was just that—an accident! God was doing some awesome work in our hearts and souls. I finally felt *free*—a new kind of freedom that I had never had before—freedom to hug my mother and love doing it and knowing that my feelings were real!

After those four weeks, I no longer harbored any ill will toward my mom nor did I feel cheated out of a life without a mother who wasn't injured. I knew that God uses everything for his good, and ours, when we turn our problems over to him. For the first time, I felt true, honest, and unhindered love for my mother.

My husband and I bought our own home soon after, but I kept very close tabs on my mom. She eventually moved in with me, my husband, and six children when my youngest son, Gabriel, was two years old, and she stayed with us for a few incredible years. Those were wonderful years for me and my children. Mother helped me to recognize the gift of song that she witnessed in my son Elijah. She is the one who suggested that he start performing with the Greater Richmond Children's Choir of which he became a member for several years, and eventually received a scholarship to perform with the choir in Japan.

My mother admitted that she continued to harbor deep guilt about how her handicap had affected our entire family. The emotional healing between my mother and me helped us to develop one of the closest and warmest relationships that any mother and daughter could have. I have learned that what is supposed to happen does. It may take a long time to face ourselves and the trials of our past, but when we do with the help of the Lord, we grow into the person God created us to be.

I have learned to be content with the family God puts me in and to find joy in it. I remember the good things in my life along with the bad, but the pain is no longer associated with the bad. My heart is free to experience the love of Christ unhindered. I thank the Lord for his patient work in my life and for healing me and for giving me a loving relationship with my mother. We can get through any pain through the power of Jesus Christ working in our lives.

I will add here, that by the time, my mom and I were finding forgiveness and healing through the sharing of our past hurts. I had forgiven my dad for the things that had happened between us. Now we are experiencing a healthy father-daughter relationship. I found that I could remember the good things that he did and the lessons that he taught us in life, that formed the strong moral standards that I live by. I respect that in him. I found love in my heart for him as a father who had also experienced pain, doing the best that he could by his own understanding. Once he stopped drinking after several years of marriage with Joyce, he became a more content person and started making amends with the family.

At the present time, my husband, Nathan, and I pastor Freedom Ministries Worldwide Inc. in Henrico County, Virginia (www.freedomministriesworldwide.org). We also have a very active ministry for the last twenty-five years in Kenya, East Africa, and neighboring countries where we have established churches and schools, as well as taking care of orphans. We have six children (Crystal, Sara, Allan, Elijah, Elisha, and Gabriel) and seven grandchildren. We are just now celebrating our thirty-fifth anniversary.

## A New Beginning

That my six-year-old daughter had felt such crippling anguish over her childish fit of anger toward me had never entered my mind. That she had carried that anguish through so many years of her young life broke my heart.

Having Susie confide those old, dark feelings to me became a much-needed catharsis for us both and served to break down all of the barriers that had kept us from sharing our deepest love with each other. I had my faith in the Lord to sustain me through all of my ordeals, but Susie had not come to the Lord until much later. She had suffered needlessly, by herself, when I could have and would have eased her dear, little heart so quickly.

After Susie and I hugged and wept together, she also told me that when Don had left for Vietnam for his one-year tour of duty, she had begun to view me as a "cool person." Susie said, "I found out that my mom was a fun person who liked to dance, draw pictures, and had always loved animals as much as I did." I believe we were all more relaxed when Don was away because, as a career military man, his parenting style was, as might be expected, very regimented. He was often very hard on the children. Don was a man who expected jobs to be done right the first time. His motto was, "If you can't take the time to do something right the first time, you sure as heck don't have time to do it a second time." Don taught the children to have strong work ethics that they have carried with them throughout their lives, and they have learned to be grateful for it.

While Don was away, the children and I finally had the freedom to collect the many different kinds of animals that made up our growing menagerie. I also taught the children how to dance, even showing them how I used to belly dance in my younger days when I was a performer.

Susie and I started to laugh remembering the many good times that we had shared. After her bold confession, she and I have grown much closer than either of us could have previously predicted. Susie and her family are a great blessing to me, and I thank the Lord for them each and every day.

## Donna's Story

I honestly don't remember much of my childhood. However, I recall that Mom asked me to help her more than she did the others. I remember doing most of the housework although we were each assigned specific weekly chores. I usually did the vacuuming, cooking, waxing, etc., because Mom said that I performed those tasks very well. I remember being scared many times, afraid that I might do something wrong that would hurt Mom unintentionally when trying to help her. I prayed and cried a lot for her. She was always so apologetic that we had to help her as much as we did, but I never minded. I cannot imagine how degrading or embarrassing it has been for my mother to accept some of the things we have had to do for her. To this day, she only prefers certain ones of us to help her with personal needs.

Most of my memories are fragmented vignettes of my family and me working and playing together.

Every week, we traveled in our station wagon to Grandma's house in Chesterfield County, and I would always fall asleep on the way there.

I remember fixing lunches for everyone in the morning and babysitting and helping with homework in the afternoon. I remember I loved to listen and dance to music. Many times I would bounce on the couch or sway back and forth while listening to my favorite songs.

I had to work hard in school since nothing seemed to come easy. But with a great deal of work, I finally got my name on the honor roll during the last couple of years in high school. I also remember that I went to two middle schools and two high schools, finally graduating from Menchville, with honors. I loved to read, and many times Dad would tell me to get outside for some fresh air because I would either be reading, doing homework, bouncing on the couch or dancing to music, or helping Mom with inside chores.

I remember that every time we moved, which was about every two years, we had a lot of cleaning, clearing away, and house fixing to do. We all worked hard as a family, but we were also scared of doing anything wrong because we would get severely reprimanded by Dad, and it seemed that every time we turned around, Momma needed us for something. We had very little leisure time, but that's what it took for us to survive as a family.

The year when Dad was in Vietnam, we all had animals: the family dog, guinea pigs, squirrel monkey, and a mynah bird. Tim had the bird (of which he found later that he was allergic) and the first word it had learned was my name. I would get mad because I would have to stop what I was doing, usually upstairs, and run to see what "Momma wanted" only to find out it was the mynah bird who had called my name. I remember one time when we were all "discussing" who mother called the most, the mynah bird answered that question for us—because it was at that moment the bird actually called *my* name. We all laughed; it truly was funny.

While Dad was gone, Momma wanted to earn extra money so she would babysit other kids; however, we children were the ones who actually took care of them by changing diapers, etc. I must admit that we worked more than we played, but sometimes it seemed that our work was our play since we all got along well together—often much better than Mom and Dad did. I remember sitting outside on the porch steps or on the house stairs brokenhearted and crying when Dad would be fighting with Momma.

Dad was gone a lot, but when he was home, our family shared a lot of activities. Dad expected a great deal from us, but I love him for staying with us and teaching us to have integrity, how to be true to our word, doing things right the first time, being the best we could be, and working together as a family. I even had to learn how to take care of a car (change tires, tune it, change oil, etc.) before I could own a car. For a graduation present, dad let me choose a car. From two cars that he had chosen, I chose a basic Chevy van, stick shift. While he was teaching me to drive, I scared him a great deal; for some reason, I had a hard time making decisions as to when to turn or how long to wait before crossing in front of someone. Generally, I would choose to cross at the last minute, and dad would say, "Are you trying to kill me?"

Within the family dynamics, there is usually what's known as a pecking order, and our family was no exception. I always felt sorry for Donny because Dad seemed to pick on him the most; I thought it was because learning did not come easy for him, and dad was not very patient. I never really knew the real reason until much later in life.

I remember the time when I was getting ready to step out the door with dad to go away to a four-year college to study in the special education field but started crying on the front porch with "bags" in hand. Dad asked me what was wrong, and I stated that I just did not feel right going away from Mom for so long. Dad, sensing my uneasiness and possibly determining in his own mind that Mom really still needed my help, made some calls to a friend who was a counselor at a community college within driving distance. I enrolled at Thomas Nelson Community College. I felt as if a big boulder had been lifted from my shoulders. I drove back and forth from home for two years, graduating with an associate degree in pre-ed. I then felt release to transfer to a four-year college to complete my special education degree. I stayed in the dorms for one year then shared an apartment with a fellow colleague who was also majoring in communication disorders. Dad paid for my tuition and residency, and I paid for my books and other necessities working my way through at a local drug store and a department store.

It was during this time that I had an accident that totaled my car. It was a cold morning around 6:30 a.m., and I was headed to Old Dominion University in Norfolk, Virginia, to do a therapy session with some students as part of an assigned clinical for my last year of bachelors in communication science as a speech therapist. I was driving my Chevy van, my first vehicle given to me by Dad. I wanted to listen to the radio to help keep me focused and more alert, but it was not working. I had a large cinderblock, which I wanted to paint and decorate, and a machete under my seat as well as a big, heavy well-supplied tool box for emergency repairs in case my van broke down. I do not remember why I had the machete—maybe to give to dad as a gift; it seems an odd thing to carry when I think back on the event of that morning. I was very tired as I had not gotten much sleep the night before. I was trying very hard to stay awake, but kept nodding off. I would roll down the window to feel the cool breeze on my face, but then the cold would get too intense, so I would roll the window back up. I tried bouncing in my seat front to back to try and stay awake and even tried singing at the top of my voice, but it was only a temporary fix. I knew that I was swerving a little, but each time I jolted back awake. As I had left the tunnel close to where I needed to get off the interstate, I had nodded off again and was jolted awake by a *thud*. Realizing that I had just run off the road onto the grassy/graveled median separating the divided highway, probably because I was still drowsy or startled, I overcompensated when I tried to turn off the median and my van careened out of control flipping over and turning around several times upside down across the road to the edge of a bridge. Thankfully I had on my seatbelt as that was the only thing holding me up. I remember praying, "Father, please save/help me? My windshield had popped out. The passenger seat had fallen down, the cinderblock, tool box, and machete were flying around, and then the van jolted to a stop. The rear door had popped open and the van had situated itself perfectly perpendicular to the rail on the bridge that kept me from falling down onto the houses below. The first thing I could think of was, "Oh no, I am going to be late for my clinic!"

The next thing I knew there were some kind people who had stopped and surrounded my vehicle to see if I was okay and had called the police. Then someone unbuckled me, and I fell down to the "top" of the van; it was a miracle that my neck had not broken as had happened with Mom. I remember asking someone to please call my clinic supervisor to let her know I would not make it to the clinic that morning and to let my roommate, Kate, know I was okay and that I would be late to class. It was a good thing I had told them to tell her that I was okay, because when she arrived at the scene she nearly freaked out by what she saw. I know that my Heavenly Father was with me that day as the only injuries I had sustained were a "knot" on my head and a bruised thumb. At the time I did not realize how fortunate I was, as my van was totaled and it was during prime time traffic. I was also deeply grateful to learn that no one else was involved or hurt. Looking back on this accident, among the several others I and my siblings and Mom have survived, it is evident that our Heavenly Father has had his angels working overtime for us. Each dramatic event has shown me that he is always there to help us and that we have no reason to live in fear as we don't leave this earth until we are called home by our Heavenly Father.

My insurance had covered the accident and I was able to buy another vehicle so that I could continue commuting to college. I graduated with a bachelor's in communication disorders from Old Dominion University and got a job as a speech therapist about forty-five minutes from home. While working, I continued my education and got my master's from Hampton University. I then worked on my clinical fellowship for a year, passed my national certification exam (on the third try—I kept missing it by two points, then finally surrendered it and my career choice to my Heavenly Father and passed with flying colors) and got certified as a speech pathologist. I was the first to graduate with a bachelor's and master's from both sides of the family; a very proud moment for us. I continue in this field to this day.

I really do not remember much else. I don't know if I have blocked out some of the painful memories of my childhood because of all that we endured after Momma's terrible accident, or if I just didn't retain things because of the concussions I sustained. I have, however, confirmation from my other siblings that they too have lost or blocked many of their own memories. I believe that trauma can alter our recall when there are things we would rather forget.

## Tim's Worst Nightmare

Tim was sixteen years old, driving my husband's 1978 Ford Country Squire station wagon for the first time. He hadn't yet qualified for his driver's license but had received a learner's permit. With the permit, according to Virginia's Department of Motor Vehicles, Tim was allowed to drive a car as long as there was an adult driver in the front seat with him.

Don, our five children, and I were in the car together returning from one of our regular visits to my parents' home in Richmond. Although it was cold outside, the car heater was turned up too high for me, and I had asked Tim to turn it down a little. Tim fumbled around with the dials on the dash, not sure where the button was located, when he lost control of the car. This is Tim's account of what happened:

> In the split second that I looked down at the dashboard, and before I could react, the road took a sharp turn to the right. I hadn't anticipated the quick turn and continued to steer straight ahead. I felt the car go over a rough patch of ground, and when I looked up, I saw that I was headed straight for a tree. I quickly tried to compensate and turned the wheel very hard to the right while I was going sixty miles per hour. The car flew to the opposite side of the

road, then back again. By that time, everyone in the car was awake.

Dad, who was sitting in the front passenger seat next to me, yelled, "Oh my God!" and tried to grab the steering wheel, but I kept trying to correct the car's trajectory by turning the wheel from side to side. Because I wasn't used to driving a car with power steering, I kept overcorrecting with each radical twist of the wheel. We all saw that it was too late to do anything, so we braced for the hit, and the car flew over an embankment toward the tree. Before the car hit the tree, I must have blacked out because I had no memory of the actual impact.

The embankment caused the car's front end to lift, slam onto and flatten the tree, causing less impact than if we had hit the tree head-on. We must have all blacked out for a brief time and woke up together. When we came to, Dad was sitting on the floor in front of the right passenger seat, and he was moaning from the pain in his back.

He had been wearing his seatbelt, so we couldn't figure out how he wound up on the floor.

I don't recall how long we had all been knocked out, but when we came to, there were people outside of the car asking if we were okay and trying to help.

I remember that my older brother, Donny, (whom you will remember had been in the car with Mom during the accident that broke her neck) panicked when he saw smoke pouring out of the car and the door next to him wouldn't open. With a rush of adrenaline, Donny slammed his arm into the side of the door and broke open the door. You can imagine how much strength that would have taken to break open a door as strong as the one on that solid old station wagon!

Everything happened so quickly; the police and ambulance came, and though we all recovered, I felt guilty for a long time because everyone in the car had sustained injuries except for me, not even bruises! Donna received a head concussion, some cuts and lacerations from broken glass, a broken collar bone, and injuries to her vertebra. Sue chipped two vertebrae in her back that rendered her unable to continue running hurdles in high school, and she eventually had to switch to shot put.

Dad's back injury was severe enough to require a stay in the hospital for a few days.

I took a deep breath before entering Dad's hospital room. I was waiting for a lecture of epic proportions from him, but he must have sensed my overpowering feelings of guilt, and instead of taking me to task over the accident, he chuckled and said, "Never mind, son. Those tires needed replacing anyway."

Mom had also sustained injuries that would require hospitalization, more surgery, and a lengthy convalescence. During impact, she had been thrust forward from where she sat in the center seat of the middle row into the front seat back where the force of impact broke her left knee. When I found out how bad Mom's injury was, I felt heartsick, and the family tried to be very gentle with me, reinforcing their belief that none of this had been my fault. They told me that I had always had a very kind heart and would never do anything to hurt another soul, much less my mother.

Perhaps the accident had not been my fault directly, but I have often wondered if a more seasoned driver would have reacted better than I did in the situation. In retrospect, neither I nor any other young, inexperienced driver should drive with so many others at risk in the car. I am grateful that we survived considering the range of other possible consequences.

I would like to say, though, that the accident has really made me a better, more conscientious driver. I don't panic behind the wheel anymore, even during occasions when someone pulls in front of me and cuts me off. On a couple of occasions over the past years when I was particularly tired after a hard day's work, I almost fell asleep at the wheel but was aware enough to safely steer my car off the road and onto the shoulder. Even then, I never panicked; I carefully steered straight and easily got myself back onto the road without injury to myself or anyone else.

I suppose the greatest impact that my mother's accident had on me was all of the hard work and tough times that we shared as a family. It also helped us grow very close and remain so over the years. I believe that our working together created in us a stronger purpose and a greater unity than we might have otherwise experienced during our growing up years. I have many fond memories of how much we loved and helped each other and stuck together, no matter what.

### Miracles happen

It was one morning, almost twenty years later; I was about twenty-seven years old, married and with two children, five and three years of age. I had left the house early in the morning, very upset about something. I had loaded my 1978 Chevrolet pickup truck with side ladders and lumber enough to build a 10 x 12 foot deck that was tied on top of the truck. While heading toward my job, driving down a three-lane boulevard with concrete dividers in the median separating three lanes on the opposite side, I was fussing at myself and hitting my steering wheel. I had heard "screaming" on my left side at a parking lot, so I had turned my head to look and see what was happening. Just at that moment, my tire had hit the concrete divider on the median, and due to the impact and standard steering, the steering wheel pulled right out of my hands. With the truck out of my control, I ran over the concrete divider and ran straight into a steel light pole that was in the middle of the dividers. I was going forty-five miles per hour at the time and was not wearing my seatbelt. My truck bent around the pole in front of my eyes and yet I had not moved; I had felt an undeniable presence pushing against my chest, holding me back to the point where I did not even move—even when I hit the light pole. This was the first miracle as I should have been thrown from the vehicle through the windshield, or at the very least, hit my head and chest, most likely with devastating effect. The second miracle was the amazing fact that not a single piece of lumber had fallen or flown off the truck at impact; they were all intact. Had they flown off the truck, there could have been a very real possibility of casualties with the other cars on the road. I knew that God was with me without a doubt. The third miracle happened while the tow-truck driver was getting my car ready for haul. He was a Christian, and we were talking and discussing my day and what had happened. He stated that he had the exact same pickup truck at his home and gave it to me! Not only was it the same make and model of my pickup, but it was in better shape than mine (before the accident). The only difference was the color; mine was green and his was blue. I have always been aware that God was with me, protecting me every day and in each situation. I believe in miracles and that God is always there helping us. He was with me in three different ways in this one accident. Just one of these accidents could have ruined and drastically changed any life, much less the several that I have had over the years. Anytime you get tired and down, just turn to Almighty God and to his Word. My favorite verse through it all is: Proverbs 3:5–6 "Trust in the Lord with all thine heart; and lean not into thine own understanding. In all thy ways acknowledge Him, and He shall direct thy paths" (King James Version).

## Donny's Long Struggle

I was eight years old, and Mom was taking me to the dentist. I didn't want to go. Things seemed normal. Suddenly, in a flash, *crash!* There seemed to be blood everywhere. I could not see except from my left eye with blood streaming down my other eye. I was in a deep state of shock although I remember seeing my mother's feet still resting on the floor board in front of the gas and brake pedals. From the steering wheel she seemed to be in an awkwardly bent, arching position lying across the seat with her arms dangling and her head almost in my lap and bleeding. I remember seeing the windshield smashed and a lot of people moving around outside. It happened so quickly.

At that moment in the chaos, I was deep in a state of shock and could not move. My eye was fixed straight ahead, but I saw everything in front of me and from my periphery. Then I heard my Mom calling my name. I could not move and neither could she, but I could hear her continue to call my name, "Donny, Donny, Donny..." She continued calling for me in a weak and frantic voice. I knew of and could feel my mother's pain, but she was more concerned to know that I was okay. I tried and tried to speak wanting to let Mom know that I was okay. I could not get the words out. I started feeling angry and hurt. Then somehow and from somewhere, I got the words out while Mom kept calling for me," Donny, Donny...," Then I said, "Mom, Mom, I am okay." I knew then that something was seriously wrong.

*Julia Dean Childress Widlacki*

## What Followed...

It was clear from the very beginning that my father blamed me for the accident. Why? Probably for the same reason that I blamed myself: If my mother hadn't been driving me to the dentist, there would have been no accident, and my father would still have enjoyed the life that he had imagined for himself and my mother.

At eight years old, I had no philosophical perspective on myself, nor what was happening inside the deepest level of my emotions, but I knew right away that I felt I was now the outcast of my family—the one who would absorb all of my father's anger against God and the universe for stealing any future joy he would have shared with my mother. I had changed too. I was no longer a happy, well-adjusted boy on the inside. I was unable to concentrate in school or remember things that I had studied. My mother thought that I had perhaps sustained a bigger injury during the accident than was apparent through normal testing, and I was sent for a CAT scan of my brain. Everything appeared normal physically, but the scars were deeper than any medical test would reveal. The tormented hateful look in my father's eyes after the accident while still in the hospital told of his feelings as he leaned over and whispered in my ear, "Why couldn't it have been you instead of her?"

My father chose hostility, anger, and eventually, alcohol, but in all fairness, he tried very hard in the beginning. He was very intelligent, extremely industrious and direct, and created different tools and items that helped my mother function with her limited abilities, but later on, he pushed her too hard. He wanted her to look and act as though she was physically normal when everything had become an ongoing struggle for her to accomplish the most menial tasks. She had difficulty even holding a fork to feed herself or a cup from which to drink—just ordinary things that we all take for granted. I felt my mother's pain. I watched her try to be stronger than she was and try harder to do things than she had the energy for. I witnessed how my father's impatience hurt her so deeply.

Although my father was now acting like a bully in so many ways to all of us, I became his target for everything that went wrong. He would seek me out scaring me when he was upset about anything, and when he did, I would receive the full onslaught of his pathological anger and frustrations.

If we three boys were chastised for a single event, the punishments were eked out in this way: Guy (the youngest) was verbally reprimanded, Tim was spanked, and I was not only spanked more severely, but the full force of my father's wrath was leveled at me; I always took more of the heat for their mistakes.

Things at home with my father never grew any easier. As my mother's struggles continued, my father grew less and less compassionate. He seemed to believe that his personal will would cause her recovery, and when that didn't work, he grew more hostile. Eventually, he wanted out of the marriage, but he stayed and often mistreated my mother with his tone, attitude, and cold demeanor.

There is possibly not a single person who could not understand how difficult this was for my father. He had to take care of personal things for my mother that humiliated her and possibly repulsed my father, but he did those things without complaint (in the beginning). My father never had the spiritual understanding or convictions that my mother grew to have very early in her life that seemed to have come to her very naturally.

No matter what difficulties she had to bear, my mother never acted with bitterness or anger, always accepting her suffering and trials with great dignity, and always believing that God would direct every footstep that she took. After many years of frustration, my father turned to alcohol and my mother turned, as always, to God. She held our growing family together with family prayer and a constant loving oversight that never failed us. However, personally, I was never fully able to regain my self-worth. I changed jobs like people change their clothes. Almost as soon as I became successful on a new job and when the boss or owners began to like me, I would quit. This pattern happened over and over again. I was in a self-sabotage cycle that caused me to destroy many golden opportunities. My father noticed this destructive pattern and brought it to my attention. I knew he was right, but I had difficulty figuring out why I was doing it and didn't understand it and felt unstable most of the time.

I joined the Navy and was doing quite well, graduating second in my Torpedoman training class. My mother flew by herself to my graduation in her condition to watch me graduate, and I was furious that my father did not come along or have someone come with her. She wanted to be present even through her struggle of moving around and having no one with her if she had fallen. It would have qualified me for duty on submarines and destroyers, but my crippled self-worth resurfaced again. During one incident, I was accused of doing something to sabotage a torpedo bay that was a malfunction of equipment and not my fault, but after the accusation had been levied against me, I told the ship's captain that I was going to leave the Navy the next time we got into port. By not defending myself properly and by creating a rash response to the accusations, I virtually ruined a good military career, and I left the service a year before my duty was up. Later on, I wrote a letter of explanation that allowed me to be exonerated, and I finally received an honorable discharge. But when I initially left the Navy, my father verbally disowned me for causing dishonor to fall upon him and his family name.

After leaving home and trying to succeed in so many jobs, I also found it very difficult to make telephone calls back to those at home. My thoughts of home caused a terrible hurtful anger to surge through me, so I stopped calling. I wanted to hear my mother's voice; I yearned to know that she was okay, and I wanted to talk to my brothers and sisters, but my conflicting emotions made it impossible to end the turmoil. I almost had to pretend to myself that I had no family in order to escape from the harsh memories of my father and my growing up years.

Since I had taken some horticulture classes in high school and loved landscaping design, I interviewed and was eventually hired as a foreman on a huge landscaping job at a new General Electric plant. I was making good money and enjoying the work, but that nagging feeling that followed me around like a second skin made me quit that job too because I was trying to escape something I felt inside me, not knowing what. So I tried commercial fishing and scalloping—thinking I could get away. I was floundering everywhere I went, and things got so bad that one night I got a six-pack of beer and drove out on the country roads toward Powhatan, Virginia, with a Buck knife on the seat next to me. My feelings of worthlessness and desolation had gotten so bad that I picked up that knife and started cutting at my wrists, but the cuts didn't do the job. I wasn't able to get the knife deep enough into my wrists to do any real damage. I must have made twelve to fifteen cuts into my wrists, but they only appeared like deep scratches. I was drinking but not drunk, and while trying to cut deeper, I ran off the road. I know now that God prevented me from taking my life that night, but the struggles weren't over. Every attempt to rebuild my own confidence only provided temporary gains. Early on, I began to exercise and body-build in an effort to gain control over some portion of my life. I even won second place in a heavy weight lifting contest for the state of Florida, but deep inside, I was still fighting for emotional survival.

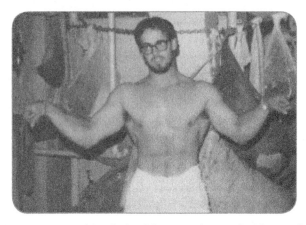

Strength training and body building made me feel less vulnerable.

Up to a certain point, everything I did was self-defeating, but slowly, gradually, I was able to begin putting together the parts of my life that needed healing. It was also during this time and when Dad first left Mom in 1986 that my wife probably saved my life, and not on just one occasion but several. My wife was nine months pregnant with our first daughter. Dad was still very distraught and angry about the way fate had plagued him, and he still had blamed me for the accident. He had called me about 10:30 in the evening and asked me to meet him alone, and I had agreed. My wife happened to overhear part of the conversation and heard the worry in my voice. When I got off the phone, my wife could tell I was troubled, and she did not want me going alone. She insisted that she come along as she sensed something was not right and that Dad was not in his right mind. When we arrived at Dad's home about 11:00 in the evening, he was sitting in a chair in his front yard with a whiskey bottle and a shot gun. When he saw that my wife was with me, he said, "Oh, you brought her with you," and he proceeded to talk with me. After looking at my wife, he had put the gun down. On another occasion, Dad called me again just before dark and specifically asked me to come alone this time. As I was getting ready to leave, my wife asked me where I was going. I told her that I was going to Dad's and he specifically asked me to come alone and to meet him by the water. My wife was emphatic that I not go alone. I did not want her to come because Dad made it a point that he wanted me to come alone. It was at this time that my wife got hysterical, and so I unwillingly let her come with me and later realized that she probably saved my life again. When we arrived at the waterfront, Dad was sitting in his car with a pistol in his hand on his lap facing the water. When I saw Dad, I got out of the car and he looked distraught. Then my wife got out of the car. My father started to react with the gun in his hand and then he saw my wife. At that point, he shook his head and looked angry and acted as though he was going to throw the pistol on the floorboard of his car but still had it in his hand and then told me, *"I told you to come alone!"* At this point, he put the pistol under a coat on the passenger side of his car. Then he said, "I do not want to talk now," and then drove off. Situations like this happened on a couple occasions, following dad's first divorce from mom. When Dad divorced Mom, it caused me to *snap,* and my anger manifested itself in my marriage, my life, and I even lost my job. It was with the love of my wife and my own two children that I began to take responsibility for my destructive behaviors, and I have now been on my last job for the past twenty years.

After my father had divorced my mother (against her will both times), he remarried a woman named Joyce and seemed to find some peace for his own life. About twenty years after the incidents with the guns, my dad found out that he had cancer. It was at this time that I reached out to forgive him and he in turn asked for my forgiveness. Throughout the course of the next couple of years, Dad asked me on several occasions while we were fishing together if there was anything I wanted him to discuss about the past. I said, "No, the past is past, and I have a relationship with you that I cherish." Dad consistently called and wanted to talk to and see me about the things he knew he had done wrong against me and the family and to develop a better relationship with me. He apologized and said he wished that he could change the past but was aware that there was no going back, only forward. Because I am a Christian and believe that I must forgive others in order to be forgiven myself, I found that I was able to forgive my father. After his brutal divorce from my mother, I don't think dad realized the full impact of his actions even when none of his children would speak to him for quite some time. Gradually, my father had apologized to each of us, and he has tried to make whatever amends he could make possible.

I now have a meaningful and grateful relationship with my father that for many, many years I had believed was impossible. There are still some hard memories that bleed through into my conscious mind, and although I am not totally recovered, I am far better off today than I have been since my mother's accident. I truly cherish the times and the relationship that I ended up having with my dad and my mother

My father has now been diagnosed with bladder cancer, and though his condition is terminal, he is managing to live out his remaining years with treatment.

In my eyes, Dad had no problem with forgiveness and ended up with a truly repentant heart. My mother has a big heart; she has been the core of our family's survival, and through Christ, she remains the only reason we have stayed strong with our faith in God. She has set the standard for her children, and we have each survived and prospered because of it. Through the years, my mother has become a source of great inspiration to everyone she meets. She is a remarkable woman, and though she has felt guilty about not being the kind of mother she wanted to be (in her own mind), she has been that mother to me, and much, much more.

I remember a very poignant episode when my mother was trying her best to exercise her parental role as disciplinarian.

I'm sure we all took some advantage of the fact that she couldn't maneuver well enough to give us a quick swat when we needed it.

My dad had fashioned a fiberglass fishing rod (spanking stick) with a big handle and rope so that Mom could hang on to it. He had made this tool for her so that she would feel she still had some control in disciplining us, which was important to her. With a tribe of five children, she needed something to gain control during those times when children need a sharp reprimand. I can still see Mom trying to spank me with the contraption, and I deserved it because I was very mischievous.

It was not the spanking that I remember as much as watching Mom struggle to spank me. I remember her frustration, hurts, and disappointment when being unable to level the rod on my behind and give me a good, needed swat. I remember watching her cry as she leaned over the counter in order to keep from falling down because she had such a hard time holding onto the stick. Watching her struggle so hard to keep control of me, her errant child, hurt deeply and made me realize again that my constant sorrow was because I felt responsible for all of my mother's suffering and pain. I developed the ability of self-preservation to turn off what I did not want to hear, even with my family because it sometimes reminded me of painful discomforting feelings or bad memories.

For a long time, I felt as though I was being cheated out of life because I had the talent and skills to become successful at anything I wanted to do but felt I never would be able to accomplish anything worthwhile because of my crippling low self-esteem that always invaded my thoughts in the form of haunting childhood memories.

Mom and Dad had also been robbed of almost everything good they had expected from life, but they had tried to persevere as best they could manage. Having my own children made me realize that I had to put all negative feelings behind me and make a living for my family. I started pulling those weeds of discontent from my thoughts—those self-defeating thoughts that promulgated low self-worth, guilt, and anger. It has been a slow process, a time of healing that has given me back my life, though some of those old memories still try to creep inside. Through my relationship with Jesus Christ, my Lord and Savior in faith, they fade out, and peace overcomes all. *Hallelujah!*

I can't say that I am totally recovered from those lost years where I was barely hanging on to life, but I have been healed emotionally from within through God's grace and have come a long way toward healing with the love of my family and by watching the heroic life of my mother who has been the truest example of courage that I have ever seen. My rainbow has been the restored relationship with my father, the heart and strength of my mother and the relationship I have with my children and wife.

## Five-Year-Old Guy Heard the Crash

Dad heard the crash from our house and hightailed it down the street toward the accident. I was only five years old and don't know how I got there, but I remember seeing a photographer on top of Mom's car taking a picture of the wreckage with my mom, brother Donny, and Dad, who was holding her head. The picture of that moment is emblazoned in my mind because I saw the worried look on Dad's face. I did not know at the time how serious the accident was. After that, the next thing I remember is when Mom came home in her walker. Grandma was at the house, and Mom came home over the weekend for the first time. It was a big deal for all of us. Aside from that, I remember the different babysitters.

One time, I was tasting a "mud pie" and the babysitter stopped me. I remember being in the back yard setting fire to the dog house with my brother Donny.

I recall many fragmented memories of those days, but as the youngest of the five children, my impressions are somewhat vague.

Later on, I remember watching my older brother Donny working out with weights. I used to make fun of him, and he said, "Instead of laughing, why don't you join me." I asked him why he wanted to work out so hard, and I won't ever forget his answer. He said, "I want to grow strong enough to protect Mom."

Although Dad had designed quite a few gizmos that would help Mom around the house and to become more independent, he refused to accept the fact that she could not regain the strength in her arms and legs that she had prior to the accident. He didn't understand how difficult everything was for her and kept repeating, "You can get better, but you're not trying hard enough." He wanted her to be whole again and could not accept the fact that her spinal injury was going to prevent that from happening.

Dad's determination to get Mom better was not only about her recovery but had a great deal to do with him feeling cheated. Dad had lost the wife (the one he married) who used to do all of the activities we had enjoyed as a family, and everything became harder on him after the accident.

Dad could be angry and mean sometimes, then caring and helpful the next. It made us all nervous when he came home and drove up the driveway because we did not know what to expect.

If we had been watching television when he came in, we were usually told to turn it off. Dad was very talented and industrious, though, and he would make us help him with his "projects," which actually helped us develop many skills that would help us later in life. I remember making things in the garage and helping Dad remodel houses.

Some of my strongest memories are those when we would go places as a family, and I would push Mom in the wheelchair. I remember people's faces as they looked at her. They seemed to look at her as though she was less of a person, which hurt my heart because nobody would ever know just how much this beautiful woman had suffered. I was determined from that time on to have a kind heart toward everyone I met. Mom always kept smiling and was so nice to people, always putting up a brave front and pretending things were all right.

Mom always tried to make things brighter for us when dad was gone to make up for the times we seemed to be nervous and upset while he was home. We loved Dad but were confused by the irrational anger he often showed toward us.

I think because some of the people in Mom's life didn't always treat her as well as she deserved, she grew to love animals as though they were her children. Mom always connected with the young and the innocent because her spirit was pure. She taught us how to care for others by caring for our pets.

These experiences taught all of us to have unconditional love for something besides ourselves.

We boys and the girls did a lot of work with dad. He taught us to develop good work ethics and skills that each one of us utilize to this day. Most importantly, we were taught to be individuals of our word.

In 1981, Dad had given each one of us $5,000 (five thousand dollars) as payment for all the years of helping him on the houses that he would buy as investments.

I was a freshman at Old Dominion University at the time and used the money to buy my first car (a Toyota Corolla). I got student loans and worked my way through college, though never finished my last year. I initially had majored in civil engineering because I wanted to be in the architect field as I love building, creating, and drawing. I was in the field for three years but had decided to switch majors to pre-med so that I could go into the field of plastic surgery. This decision was a direct result of what I had gone through following a serious accident where I was severely burned.

The accident happened while I was sleeping in the upstairs bedroom of a rented home in Norfolk, Virginia. My roommate, a pizza deliveryman who kept late hours, came home and started watching TV and smoking cigarettes downstairs. He started feeling groggy and finally went upstairs to bed.

About an hour later, he awoke to the noise of fire crackling somewhere downstairs.

He yelled, "House is on fire!" and then ran outside and across the street to call the fire department—*but* I thought he was playing a prank, and I went back to sleep. Soon after, I awoke and saw smoke all around me, and I could hardly breathe. I rushed downstairs just as an explosion occurred that caused the glass panes in the living room to burst. When this happened, the oxygen rushed inside the house causing the flames to get bigger. I was immediately covered in glass and fire, and in such horrific pain that I became frozen from shock before the realization came clear to me that I was probably going to die. I ran for the place where I thought the front door was but couldn't see anything except pitch black and glowing embers. Because my roommate had closed the door behind him when he ran out, I smacked right into it. The flesh of my upper arm stuck and fused to the door, burning the skin off my upper arm. I managed to reach for the door handle, which was fiery hot, blistering my hand as soon as I touched it. I kept hold of it and turned the handle while the flames were roaring around me and filling my lungs with black smoke. By that time, I was out the door with my hair smoking and fire all around me. I thought my roommate was still inside the house so I continued to yell his name. Just as I was ready to run back inside the house and help him, I heard him call my name from across the street.

I was taken to the hospital with second- and third-degree burns and was there for six days during which I spent much of the time in the saline baths. The doctors also had cut the burnt skin from my arm, hand, and sides of my face next to my temples. As I was being treated in the saline tank, I saw all of the other injured people and understood their suffering because of what I was going through; it was the worst pain I had ever experienced. My heart reached out to them and wanted to do something to help stop their suffering.

My desire to help people mainly came from growing up with Mom, but this experience led me toward wanting to major in plastic surgery. After investigating that career field with actual plastic surgeons, I was told that the worst aspect of the field was the frivolous lawsuits that caused medical insurance costs to soar. My career choices have changed a couple of times over the years, but what remains—the most important message I can share with anyone—is that nothing happens by accident.

While going to college in Norfolk, Virginia, I worked two jobs: one of them was as at Smalls' Tru Value Hardware Store, and the other was at Milton's.

One day, while I was working my shift at Milton's as one of the store managers, I received a phone call from my other boss at Tru Value asking if I could install a ceiling fan for a customer who wanted to surprise her husband with it for his birthday. He gave me the number to call her. I spoke with the woman and had offered to put up the fan at a later time when I got off from work, but she insisted that she wanted it to be installed right then so the fan would be in place as a surprise to her husband when he came home from work. As I was discussing this on the phone, my good friend Bill, who was also a shift manager at Milton's, came into the store and had overheard my conversation. Bill said he understood my predicament and offered to fill in for me.

I asked him whether he was sure, and he confirmed that he didn't mind helping me out because he had nothing else going on at the time. Little did I know that this was another life-changing experience.

While I was away installing the ceiling fan, there had been a robbery at the Milton's store. To my shock and horror, the robber had taken the life of my good friend Bill. I was devastated and left with a nagging feeling of guilt because it should have been me who had died, not my friend.

I had gone back to my apartment to clean up before going back to Milton's, and when I walked in the door, my roommates looked at me as though I were a ghost. They had been watching a live newscast on television about the robbery at Milton's and that the manager, Guy Widlacki, had been killed. Just then my phone rang, and it was mom; she was frantic because she had been watching the same newscast. I told her that I was okay but that I had to go. I hung up the phone and sprinted all the way to Milton's. I had to explain to the police that I was not dead, and sadly, I had to identify my friend Bill, who was dead and lying on the floor.

Apparently, Bill did not have any identification on his person, and all the police had to go by was the plaque on the wall that named the manager on duty, which was supposed to have been me.

Identifying Bill's body was one of the hardest things I have ever had to do.

Mom always told me that an angel saved me that day, but I still felt guilty because Bill died in my place.

Ever since 2003, Mom has been living with me and has been a constant support for me and my two children. She almost always has a positive attitude and looks on the bright side of things with a spiritual day-to-day appreciation. She does not discuss the constant pain and difficulty she endures; she just keeps on going, trying always to make the best of things. She is and has been an inspiration for us all.

My mother begins each day new as if to say, "I am up, so what do I need to do today?" Without Mom, I do not know where I would be today—possibly dead. My mother has also been a great inspiration for my two wonderful children, Shaye and Valen. She is an ongoing positive influence in their lives as she has always been in mine.

As a single father, I am glad my mother is living with me because my children have the opportunity to witness an example of what a good mother is and should be. I want them to know this is how I was raised, and this is what I want for them.

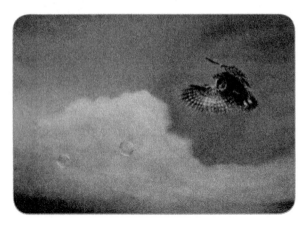

*Illusions of Life*, painting by Guy Widlacki at www.guywidlacki.com

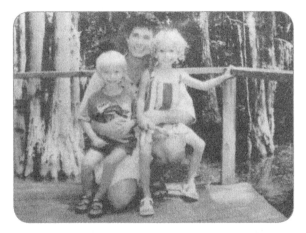

Guy holding his son, Valen, and daughter, Shaye

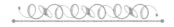

# Don's View

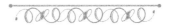

There is no way that I can speak for my ex-husband, Don, and convey the complexity of his own struggles and emotional responses to our difficulties after my accident. In all fairness to him and how he endured those difficult years, I would like to include the interview that Don recently shared with our daughter, Donna.

I believe reading Don's words will enable my readers to gain some insight into Don's strengths. It will better illustrate the many fine traits, values, and character that Don brought to our marriage and taught to our children: to become the strong, independent, resourceful, and caring individuals they are today.

I do not renege or retract any statements I have made in these pages regarding the difficultly of our marriage following my accident, but I want my readers to understand what Don also endured, and that enables me to forgive him. I wonder how many husbands could have endured all that he went through for so many years. I will always be grateful that Don helped and supported me and our children at great sacrifice to his own happiness for as long as he could manage to do so.

## The Interview with Dad by Donna Hepner

Dad was a survivor. He left his home in Chicago before the age of eighteen years old. He was able to find work because he looked older than he was. Dad told me that his family had "nothing" during his growing up years, so to him, our struggling family was, in comparison, "doing all right." We had a roof over our heads and running water, "What more do you want?" he would say. Dad was a very proud man and would not take handouts. When we lived in Greenville, Mississippi, two ladies came to our house with a couple of bags of food, saying, "We understand that you're having a little trouble." But dad said we were doing just fine, and they should take the food to a family that really needed it.

Dad believed that no matter what was broken, he could fix it. We always had "clunker cars" as he would call them. He would buy a car for $100–$150 and fix it with his friend Bob Webster, a good mechanic. Dad would then drive it hard until it died and then get another one.

When we lived in Converse, Texas, our house was situated atop a steep hill. At the time, Dad owned an old WWII Willys Jeep that wouldn't start most of the time. The only way he could rely on getting the car moving during those times was to park at the top of the hill, turn the key, take off the brake, push on the clutch, and pop it while going down the hill. When he was at work, he would ask his buddies to push the jeep from behind to help get it started. Dad endured this hardship because he didn't have enough money to get the car fixed. He had learned early in life to make do with whatever life presented without whining about it.

As each of us children graduated from high school, Dad bought us a good but cheap used car that was mechanically sound and gave it to us as a graduation present. We had no choice as to the type of car he picked for us, but at least we got one! Mine was an old Volkswagen van that was a stripped down, stick shift model, but it drove well. We all had to learn how to take care of a car before we were allowed to have one (including changing tires, tune ups, changing oil, etc.).

I recall a time when I told dad that my car didn't sound right, and he said it sounded like the carburetor, so I went to the store and bought an overhaul kit. According to Dad, I had taken the entire carburetor apart and placed each piece in an orderly fashion on his work bench. When he saw what I had done, he thought, *Oh no!* but he left me alone to figure it out. After I had finished, he said that I put it all back together, and it worked like new. He was very proud of me and very surprised that I had done the job by myself. Looking back now, I am very grateful to dad for not doing things for us but teaching us to be independent and trying to figure things out for ourselves.

Dad joined the Navy on August 16, 1954, and worked on high-speed diesels that propelled the ships. His job was to stand inside them and test their performance. He also ran the liberty launch boat that held about fifty men/troops, which brought them back and forth from the ship to land. This was an extra job although without extra pay. Dad loved the Navy but decided to leave when his stint was up in order to spend more time with Mom and us children.

He decided to join the Air Force but regretted losing the two stripes he had earned while in the Navy. He entered the Air Force as an E3, but he had made the decision that our family was more important to him than money.

While he was in the Air Force, Dad worked as a jet engine mechanic and enjoyed his job. He especially enjoyed taxiing the jets on the runway in order to figure out what was wrong with them and rechecking them to see whether he and his crew had correctly identified and fixed the problem. Dad said that after he had worked at that job for about six months, an "idiot" staff sergeant actually took one of the planes up in the air, and after that only the pilots could taxi the planes. Dad said that even though he wore earplugs, he had lost a lot of hearing for some high-frequency sounds, but he could hear low frequencies.

Dad enjoyed working in the Air Force but didn't like the twelve-hour shifts, seven days a week, without extra pay, and that also kept him away from the family more than he had expected.

Dad progressed in the Air Force to the rank of E5 staff sergeant on October 1, 1964, and E6 technical sergeant on September 1, 1968. As the family was growing, Dad was not home much as he had to take on extra jobs because he was hungry, had a family to feed, and was a fast learner who would do whatever work there was to do. Dad did not want a large family because he wasn't able to spend the one-on-one quality time that he wished to give us when he came home from work. All of us would come to him for attention at the same time. He believed that Mom wanted a big family (and would have had more children had Dad not gotten a vasectomy while serving in Japan). Dad felt that we gave Mom a sense of belonging and filled her need to give and receive unconditional love.

Dad was very good at whatever he did; he was a hard worker, had great common sense, and learned quickly. He would often take on another eight-hour job, not telling his boss that he was also working for the military. Dad would stay with each job for about three months until he was too worn out and had to quit. He worked as an electrician machinist in a machine shop, taped and stacked boxes in a cardboard factory, made neon signs at a neon sign company, to name a few. Most of the places he held part-time jobs wanted him to stay and would offer him raises, but Dad would always say that he was moving out of the area. Dad would rest up while working at home, making some things to sell. He did this on and off for many years after he and Mom were married.

When Dad wasn't working an extra job, he designed and made leather goods for sale (my favorite is a small hand-tooled leather purse that I still have to this day). He was very meticulous with his work and kept at each piece until it was "just right." He also made framed pictures by placing a selected picture on a thick piece of flattened oak, pine, or cherry wood; chiseling and carving sections of wood around the picture, and then shellacking the picture and frame. We had several of his works of art hanging around our home as we were growing up.

When dad was stationed in San Antonio, Texas, we lived in a rented farmhouse from a nice, black farmer. When he asked Dad how he felt about renting from a black man, Dad said, "I don't care if you're pink." Dad said that the owner liked the answer, and they got along fine. The farmer even paid for the heat whose source was a single, leaky, propane heater that was situated in the middle of the house.

One time, the farmer asked Dad if he could turn down the heat as it was costing more than the rent he was charging for the house. Dad told him that he just couldn't do that because it was still cold even with the heat turned up and reminded him that he had also been fixing up the place better than he had found it. (While living there, dad owned a table saw that he used to make items to sell and would fix up things in the house just because it needed fixing.) The farmer no longer mentioned the cost of heat.

Dad saved a lot of money because he had the skills to fix things that broke at home; he was an all-around handyman.

Most of our vacations were annual camping trips that we enjoyed as a family. Dad may have been mean at times, and he was often a tough task master, but he had a high degree of integrity and always kept his word—a character trait that we all learned early on about him. Whatever he said, he meant, and whatever he said he would do, he did. This was an important value that each one of us put into practice.

Dad always said he and Mom were "just kids raising kids," and at times didn't know where to "draw the line" when it came to our discipline. He was a hard but loving father and did not know any other way to raise us. Mom and Dad did the best that they could manage.

## The Accident (from Donna's Interview with Dad)

On that fateful day, Mom had asked Dad to drive Donny to the dentist because she was tired, but Dad said that he was also "beat." Although she didn't feel like going, Mom decided to take Donny to the dentist anyway because their dentist was usually booked, and they would have had to wait quite a while for another appointment.

It was already dark when Mom was driving Donny back home from the dentist appointment. Just as she was making a left-hand turn onto our street, out of apparently nowhere, headlights appeared coming straight at our car. A couple of teenagers ran through a red light and hit the driver's side of our car broadside.

Because the accident had happened only a block and a half from our house, Dad had heard the crash and felt an intuitive nudge that he had better go and see what had happened. He ran out the front door, and when he got only a few yards from the accident, he saw that it was our family car that had been hit—and hit badly!

Dad ran to the car window on the driver's side, and when Dad saw Mom's condition, he could hardly comprehend her injuries and the devastation at the scene. He was in a state of shock and disbelief but quickly took the place of the stranger who had been holding Mom's head so that she could breathe.

The police came, a newspaper photographer came, and finally, the ambulances arrived that took Donny to the air base hospital, and Mom to the local hospital where she needed more extensive care.

Dad hitched a ride to the hospital every day to see and feed Mom, then hitched another ride to go see Donny who had sustained some minor cuts and a concussion. When Dad saw Donny, he was lying in bed with a bandage over his head and was still in shock. Dad said that Donny looked up at him with eyes the size of saucers and said that he wanted to go home. The base commander allowed Donny to go home and drove him and Dad back to the house.

A man showed up at the house introducing himself as a lawyer and asked Dad if he could represent the family regarding the accident. Dad said, "Okay, I guess." As it turned out, the kids driving the other car only had $10,000 in insurance and the lawyer took $5,000 of it for his services. Dad was very upset with the lawyer because he was not ethical by taking so much, especially since the case never went to court, and it was settled quickly. Dad used that money to get another car, and the remainder was spent trying to help Mom and the family.

At the hospital, Dad said he got very angry at the doctor who said, in front of Mom, that she would never be able to walk or use her arms again.

Dad pushed the doctor out of the room and said, "How dare you say that in front of my wife!" Dad said the remark was cruel and insensitive. That particular doctor never came back.

Dad was determined and angry. After a couple of weeks, the nurses and doctors permitted Dad free rein in the hospital, and visiting hours no longer applied to him. Dad came to the hospital every day to feed Mom, and every time he saw her, he would go home and do a lot of praying, crying, and begging. He would tell Mom, "You are going to walk and use those hands again because I cannot handle our five children by myself."

I believe that Don's interview with Donna will illustrate his perspective and offer my readers an idea of his strengths, his endurance, and his character that helped our family survive during the difficult years following my accident. Don is a fine man whose life was impacted as deeply as was my own, and I hold no hard feelings toward him for having to find his own happiness after suffering through so many years of hardship, on so many levels.

*Rainbows After the Storms*

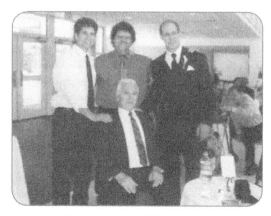

*Back row,* Guy, Tim, and Donny; *seated,* Don

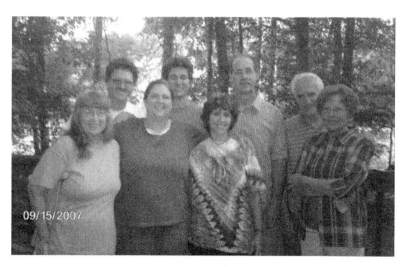

Family photo
*Front row:* Me (far left) Susie, Donna, Joyce
(ex-husband Don's wife at far right end)
*Back row:* Tim (left) Guy, Donny, my ex-husband, Don (right)

Time does indeed have a way of healing old wounds. Even though Don and my five children were raised with a heavy hand when it came to discipline, each one of them has admitted gaining benefits from learning how to be self-reliant from their father's example.

# And Now...

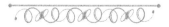

I am currently classified as a walking quad. You are probably asking what that means. It is someone who is still paralyzed in all four limbs but can still walk. I have recently learned that I am one of fifty-six walking quadriplegics (of record) in the nation. I use my wheelchair if I have to go out anywhere for any length of time, and I still need help but try to manage the best that I can. I am still paralyzed internally and still, on occasion, have bowel accidents.

I still don't have any feeling from my chest down, nor do I feel itching sensations, or hot and cold water (except on my hands). I am in constant visceral pain, but I experience no sensation of pain on the outside of my body. I walk very slowly with the aid of crutches; if I fall, I cannot get up without someone's help. My hands still do not function normally, but I am still able to dress and bathe myself in a sit-down shower. I stay very weak, but by God's grace, I make it through each day. During the last eight years, I have had numerous operations, among which was a surgically placed permanent catheter.

I have gone to an orthopedic doctor to find out why my arm had been growing very weak and hurting constantly. The diagnosis was that my rotator cuff had been completely torn in half, and because of several complications, the doctor could not perform corrective surgery. I praise God, though, that I am still able to use my arm well enough to bathe and dress myself. It is a miracle in itself that I can use my right arm and hand.

The neurosurgeon that I go to in Norfolk does not want me to walk with crutches. She has advised me to use my wheelchair instead, because she's afraid that overusing the crutches might cause me more lasting harm. I suppose I am a bit stubborn, but I still prefer to use my crutches. After everything I've been through, I don't want to completely lose the ability to walk.

My wonderful children are always there to help me as I need them.

## Living with My Youngest Son

Since 2003, I have been living with my youngest son, Guy, who invited me to live with him and my beautiful grandchildren, Valen and Shaye, after his divorce. Guy has been a wonderful support throughout these years and has had to take me to the emergency room many times, often in the middle of the night.

Sometimes I wonder why in the world things happen the way they do. Guy has taken charge of my care with such a loving heart while dealing with many of life's difficulties as a single father. He even changes my catheter bag quite frequently and does so many things for me that I honestly could not manage without his help.

I almost died during a visit to the hospital emergency room this past year when I had broken out with a rash over my entire body and was going into autonomic dysreflexia, from which I could have died. (So many doctors do not believe that I could have that problem because I can walk.)

Guy had to insist that my catheter had a blockage and that it needed to be replaced so that my distended bladder could drain. Guy knew my history and immediately recognized the problem, but the doctor wouldn't listen until Guy took him by the shirt and told him, in no uncertain terms, to change my catheter so that it could drain properly. Once my catheter was drained of over 1,600 cc's of urine, I was all right again. Once again, my son saved my life. The doctors were a little shocked but did not want to admit they had gotten it wrong. One of the doctors did, however, turn to Guy and thanked him for being so persistent.

I believe doctors should be willing to listen more carefully to patients. I have had many such episodes but have managed to get through every one of these by God's grace. I should do in-service training sessions with doctors on the subject of walking quads. The only doctor whom I have found who knows about this situation is the emergency room doctor in Portsmouth.

I will be starting a program in March 2012 with a certified therapy training center in Carrollton, Virginia, run by Patty Allen, that assists dog owners who wish to participate in a program that will train their pet to become a certified therapy dog.

I will be taking my little dog, Angel, to the class once a week for six weeks (with the help of Guy or Donna) to prepare Angel to pass the required test to become a certified therapy dog. Angel can then be taken to visit nursing homes, independent living facilities, and hospitals to brighten up the days for patients confined to facilities where they are unable to leave or have their own pets.

I sometimes think about the days when I was young and as free as the wind, riding my horses through the countryside. The following are pictures that I drew as I remembered those days, and though I don't lament what cannot be changed, I sometimes find myself back there, innocent of what lay ahead.

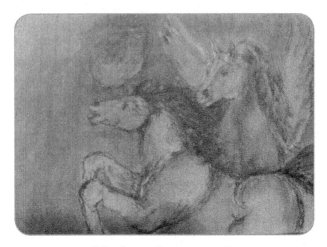

My dream horses can fly

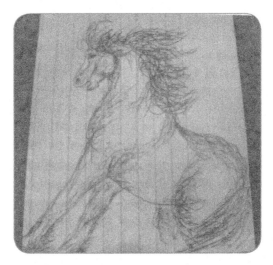

I still think of my horses and love to draw pictures of them.

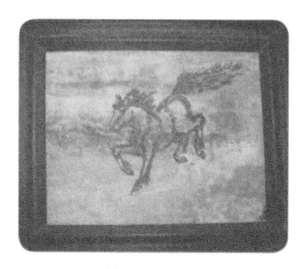

## My Vision

As I come to the conclusion of my story, I would like to add a dream vision that I had in the middle of May 2012. I believe it was a prophetic dream that the Lord gave me.

My family and I were driving in our car on a scenic road when all of a sudden, the beauty of the landscape disappeared, and in its place we saw a huge, scary pit where machines were digging out everything from inside the pit. One of the machines turned over, and I saw a man scrambling for his life. In the next instant, I saw a huge snake with a box-shaped head suddenly grab the man and gobbled him up. After that, things quickly changed, and the snake started to come after me and my family. The scene changed, and everything became white; I had a strong feeling that I had seen into hell, and I began to shout to everyone, "Get up higher! Get up higher!"

I felt an incredible urgency to get up higher so that the snake could not touch us.

As I contemplated this vision, I began to realize that the Lord is telling us all to "get up higher."

The Lord is coming back soon to take us home with him. No matter how many difficulties we face as time moves on, we will overcome if we put our trust in God.

It is my prayer that everyone will finally realize that God has each of us in the palm of his hands. I know that God will see me through any and all difficulties that may arise, and he will do the same for each of you. Our Lord Jesus will never leave nor forsake any of us.

I leave you with my heartfelt prayer that you will find your greatest blessings in life through faith in our Lord and Savior as I have. And remember, Dear Readers, do as the Lord admonishes in Galatians 6:9 (St Jerome's Catholic Study Bible), "Be not weary in doing good works." We are reminded that in the proper time, we will reap a just harvest if we *do not give up*.

Remember there is always a rainbow after the storm. God bless you all.

—Julia Dean Childress Widlacki

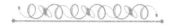

# Epilogue

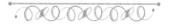

My tragedy has been turned into victory and triumph in the Lord. He has filled me with his grace and love. I give God the glory forever.

Praise God in all situations, and sincerely seek him with all your heart; he will never fail you. Our Lord is coming back, and he is calling all of us.

Know that nothing is impossible with God. Just believe and never give up, knowing that he is always with you. Be quick to forgive others so that your prayers will not be hindered. Always pray for everyone and walk in love. I pray God's blessings will be on everyone who reads my story; I pray that knowing the trials and tribulations that I have gone through—and overcome, by the grace of God—will help you in your own time of need and will help you overcome each of your trials.

Remember to give God praise in every situation, for he will justify your suffering in the end. Pray and walk with peace in his everlasting love.

My favorite scripture, Proverbs 3:5–6 gives us hope through his great promise: "Trust the Lord with all your heart, lean not upon your own understanding, in all of your ways acknowledge

Him and He shall direct your paths." (Saint Jerome's Catholic Study Bible).

Remember, he is always with you. Believe and always seek the Lord with all your heart; he will never fail you.

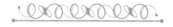

# Don's Passing

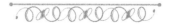

Don Widlacki
Jan. 19, 1937–Dec. 7, 2012

Don Widlacki, Julia's former husband of thirty-three years, passed away on December 7, 2012, at 5:30 a.m. at the age of seventy-five from an aggressive form of cancer that had metastasized to his liver and esophagus. To the surprise of his family, a recent bladder biopsy showed that the cancer was in remission. Don's passing was bittersweet as it happened within four days after the family found out that the cancer had just spread to different parts of his body. Thankfully, good-byes were said before Don's passing with visits from his three sons, Donny, Tim, and Guy (along with their families), Susie's son and daughter, Allen and Sara, as well as Sara's children. Don's daughters Sue and Donna were unable to be at his side when he died but were grateful to have spent time with him prior to their three-week service mission to Africa and were able to speak with him on the phone twice while there. At Don's side when he passed was his current wife, Joyce, and his grandson, Allan.

A family backyard memorial was held for Don at his home where he was remembered through family stories and anecdotes about his life. As he loved the Navy, it was decided that Don be honored with a Naval burial at sea in recognition of his distinguished service to both the Navy and Air Force.

Don Widlacki will be missed by family and friends.

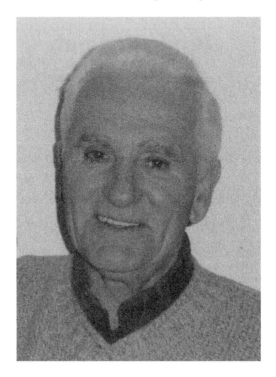

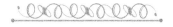

# Appendix

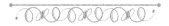

I would like to share a few words with my readers in hopes that they will encourage you as they have me throughout my life.

In my opinion, if you can do the following nine things, you can live a fulfilled life:

1 - Think
2 - Dream
3 - Laugh
4 - Cry
5 - Forgive
6 - Love
7 - Pray
8 - Hope
9 - Persevere

I always start each day with enthusiasm and communion with my God.

I try to fill each day with dreams, kindness, forgiveness, and love.

I always have hope; I thank and praise my Lord for all things each and every day.

I have learned that you should never quit or give up no matter what obstacles lie before you in life.

Life is too short not to make the best of it.

Laugh and sing and always have hope.

I hope this book has been an inspiration to you. May God bless you richly and give you grace to face what comes your way each day.

Remember
God's Mercy Endures
Forever

You may contact me through
my e-mail address: hepner38@gmail.com.

CPSIA information can be obtained at www.ICGtesting.com
Printed in the USA
BVOW06s1850010216

435062BV00017B/141/P